D0298404

#17

THE
ANTIMICROBIC
SUSCEPTIBILITY
TEST:
Principles
and Practices

With chapters contributed by:

Paul D. Hoeprich, M.D. (Chapter 3)
Professor of Medicine and Pathology
Chief, Section of Infectious and Immunologic Diseases
Departments of Internal Medicine and Pathology
School of Medicine
University of California
Davis, California

Michael A. Saubolle, B.S. (Chapter 11)
Research Associate
Section of Infectious and Immunologic Diseases
Department of Internal Medicine
University of California
Davis, California

The ANTIMICROBIC SUSCEPTIBILITY TEST: Principles and Practices

ARTHUR L. BARRY, Ph.D., MT (ASCP)

Director, Microbiology Laboratories
University of California, Davis–Sacramento Medical Center
Sacramento, California

and

Associate Professor in Clinical Microbiology
Departments of Internal Medicine and Pathology
School of Medicine
University of California
Davis, California

LEA & FEBIGER • *Philadelphia, 1976*

Library of Congress Cataloging in Publication Data

Barry, Arthur L.
  The antimicrobic susceptibility test.

  1. Micro-organisms, Effect of drugs on. 2. Drugs Testing. I. Title. [DNLM: 1. Microbial sensitivity tests—Laboratory manuals. 2. Anti-infective agents— Pharmacodynamics—Laboratory manuals. QW25 B279A]
QR69.A57B37 1976   615'.1   76-18846
ISBN 0-8121-0530-3

Published in Great Britain by Henry Kimpton Publishers, London

PRINTED IN THE UNITED STATES OF AMERICA

Print Number: 4   3   2   1

*Dedicated
to my loved ones:*
DIANE
Karen
Kathy
Bill
Brian

PREFACE

Three primary responsibilities of the clinical microbiologist are (1) to help guide the proper collection of specimens from patients showing clinical signs of infection, (2) to examine the specimens in order to identify the most probable etiologic agent(s) as rapidly and efficiently as possible, and (3) to perform appropriate *in vitro* studies that will help the physician select the most appropriate chemotherapeutic agent or combination of agents. The third area of responsibility — antimicrobic susceptibility testing — is the subject of this monograph. It was written for the laboratorian who wishes to better understand his or her role as an important member of the team responsible for the care of patients with infectious diseases. Emphasis is placed upon the basic principles by which the laboratory data are developed and applied to the clinical management of infected patients. For each type of test procedure, theoretical considerations are presented in order to explain the importance of standardization of each step and to better understand the consequences of altering each step in a standardized procedure. Although most procedures are described in sufficient detail to permit an informed technologist/microbiologist to develop an acceptable test protocol, we have tried to avoid the temptation to present a classic "cookbook" outline of each type of test described.

Procedural details are outlined to describe those techniques that are currently accepted as standard methods. In addition, suggestions are made for alternative methods for handling special situations for which the standard methods may not be adequate. These suggestions are not all firmly based upon an abundant amount of experimental data; in fact, there are often conflicting data that reflect differences of opinion and the absence of valid comparative studies. All the techniques outlined in the following pages are subject to change as new information becomes available and improved technology is developed. This monograph should be viewed as an attempt to describe the current "state of the art" for antimicrobic susceptibility testing.

To help those who may be interested in searching for additional information, we have included at the end of each chapter a list of the references consulted in preparation of that chapter. This is not intended to represent an exhaustive review of literature, and we acknowledge the fact that some significant contributions may have been omitted in our effort to conserve space.

I am especially indebted to Drs. Paul D. Hoeprich and John C. Sherris for the constructive criticism offered in reviewing portions of this manuscript. I also wish to acknowledge the invaluable assistance of Dr. Anthony K. Knirsch, who generously provided most of the data summarized in Chapters 10 and 15. A special note of gratitude is due to Miss Sandra Lindgren for her invaluable help in preparation of the manuscript.

Davis, California   Arthur L. Barry

CONTENTS

Section II. ANTIMICROBIC DILUTION TESTS

Section IV. AGAR DIFFUSION TESTS

Section I

GENERAL PRINCIPLES OF ANTIMICROBIAL SUSCEPTIBILITY TESTING

Chapter **1**

INTRODUCTION

The concept of specific antimicrobial chemotherapy was developed long before the widespread use of antibiotics in the treatment of infectious diseases. The sulfonamides were used to a limited extent before 1940, at which time the now famous Oxford group succeeded in isolating a relatively pure and stable form of penicillin. This achievement pointed out the potentialities of antibiotic therapy, which, in turn, stimulated the interest of research workers in a variety of disciplines. Major progress in the field of antibiotic chemotherapy occurred with the development of methods for mass production of high-quality penicillin, the discovery of streptomycin and later of the "broad-spectrum" and "limited-use" antibiotics, and the development of methods for production of the semi-synthetic antibiotics and synthetic antimicrobial agents.

It became obvious early that certain strains of bacteria demonstrated a high degree of resistance to each newly developed drug. Widespread use of the antibiotic tended to select the resistant variant, and after a drug had been in use for some time, resistant strains were so common that the susceptibility of a given isolate could not be predicted on the basis of previous experience with other strains of that species. For that reason it became necessary to test each isolate from individual patients in order to determine whether the etiologic agent was resistant to the antimicrobial agents available for use. The generic term "antimicrobic susceptibility tests" describes the various types of *in vitro* techniques that can be used to determine susceptibility or resistance of individual isolates. The purpose of this monograph is to review the general principles of the various laboratory techniques that can be used for evaluating the *in vitro* activity of antimicrobial agents, in order to guide the specific therapy of patients with infectious diseases.

Before progressing further, it may be well to define the terms that are commonly used in describing antimicrobial chemotherapeutic agents.

The term "chemotherapeutic agent" refers to any compound that may be administered to a patient to treat or to control a disease. The term is often applied to drugs that are selectively active against microbial pathogens and cancer cells as opposed to normal host tissues.

The term "anti-infective agent" refers to compounds that inhibit pathogenic microorganisms causing an infectious process. It implies no activity against commensal or saprophytic microorganisms.

The term "antibiotic" describes a chemical substance produced by one organism that in low concentrations is capable of inhibiting the growth of another microorganism. A very large number of antibiotics have been identified, but only a few can be used as chemotherapeutic agents since most are also toxic to the host being treated.

The term "antimicrobic" ("antimicrobial agent") may be used to designate "any substance of natural, semi-synthetic, or synthetic origin that inhibits or kills free living, commensal or pathogenic microorganisms while causing little or no injury to the host."[10]

GENERAL METHODS FOR SUSCEPTIBILITY TESTING

In his original description of penicillin, Fleming described an agar diffusion test (ditch-plate test) that was popular for many years and that has survived innumerable modifications.[8] Fleming also used a broth dilution test that, with some minor alterations, is now a widely accepted technique. In principle, the two types of susceptibility tests used by Fleming are still commonly used for testing the activity of an antimicrobic against a microorganism; however, the actual test procedures have become increasingly sophisticated and are now well standardized. With both types of susceptibility tests, the microorganism is exposed to decreasing concentrations of the antimicrobial agent, and then, after appropriate incubation, the lowest concentration that exerts an inhibitory activity is determined.

Agar Diffusion Test. A nutrient agar plate is inoculated and the antimicrobic diffuses from a reservoir into the agar medium. As the microorganisms grow, they are exposed to a continuous gradient of decreasing concentrations of antimicrobic at increasing distances from the reservoir. The reservoir can be formed by filling a ditch or a well cut from the agar plate, by filling a cylinder placed onto the agar surface, or by applying filter-paper discs that contain the antimicrobial agent. Although the methods for applying the antimicrobic differ, the principle of all agar diffusion tests is the same: the larger the zone of inhibition, the greater the degree of susceptibility of the test organism, all other variables being equal. Generally, agar diffusion tests are used only for qualitatively distinguishing between susceptible and resistant strains, but they may be standardized to provide more nearly quantitative information.

Antimicrobic Dilution Test. For quantitative estimates of antimicrobic activity, dilutions of the antimicrobial agent may be incorporated into broth or nutrient agar and then inoculated with a standardized suspension of the test organism. The adjectives "broth," "tube," "agar," and "plate" are often added to the term "dilution test" to describe the way in which the antimicrobic dilution is prepared. Such terms are actually misnomers because it is the antimicrobic rather than the broth or agar that is being diluted; clearly, the tubes or plates are not being diluted. The term "microdilution" refers to a broth dilution test that is carried out in small volumes (0.1 ml).

After appropriate incubation, the minimal inhibitory concentration (MIC) is determined as the lowest concentration that will inhibit growth of the microorganism. The MIC is generally expressed as micrograms (μg or mcg) per ml, international units (IU) per ml, or micromoles (μ moles) per ml. The tests are usually limited to doubling dilution steps and thus an MIC of x μg/ml usually means that the microorganism is inhibited by x μg/ml but is not completely inhibited by $\frac{1}{2}$ x μg/ml. The minimal lethal concentration (MLC) may be determined by transferring to an antimicrobic-free medium an aliquot of material from those tubes showing no growth. This transfer will reduce the concentration of antimicrobic by dilution and any microorganisms that were inhibited but not "killed" will be able to grow. When the test organism is bacterial, the lethal activity may be referred to as bactericidal effect; if a fungus is being tested, the MLC expresses fungicidal activity; if a viral agent is being tested, the MLC is viricidal; if *Mycobacterium tuberculosis* is being considered, the lethal end-point is tuberculocidal.

Both agar diffusion and antimicrobic dilution techniques can be extremely precise and accurate analytical methods if proper attention is paid to the technical details that are outlined in the following chapters.

STANDARDIZATION OF SUSCEPTIBILITY TESTS

Originally, susceptibility tests were described with few details concerning the many technical aspects that can influence the test results. Each laboratory worker developed a test system that seemed to fit his own particular needs, often without adequately documenting the accuracy or precision of the procedure. Consequently, numerous variations of each type of susceptibility test were being used in different laboratories. Some methods were carefully developed; others were grossly inadequate or unreliable. Since much of the routine susceptibility testing has been based on insecure foundations and different decisions on test conditions and interpretations have been made by different persons, it is not surprising that the same strain will give markedly different results when tested in different laboratories. Day-to-day variability within the same laboratory can be rather remarkable, especially if the test procedure has not been carefully defined in all details and if the test protocol is not strictly followed. As a result of these problems, many workers have urged the development of standardized methods that can be used for routine testing or at least as standard reference methods which can be used as a guide for evaluating other techniques.

In 1960, an international group of experts on antibiotics was formed to study the problem for the World Health Organization (WHO). The need for standards and some general guidelines to be followed were outlined in the Second Report of the Expert Committee on Antibiotics.[12]

Following this report, an ad-hoc group of interested persons from different countries was formed under the chairmanship of Dr. Hans Ericsson, with the sponsorship of the WHO. The group undertook a series of studies to define reference procedures that could provide a basis for comparisons of different methods. In 1971, the conclusions and recommendations of this International Collaborative Study (ICS) were published by Ericsson and Sherris.[5] Their report proposed standard reference methods for antimicrobic dilution techniques. Broth dilution and agar dilution methods were developed so that the two procedures gave nearly comparable results.

The agar dilution method was preferred because it demonstrated somewhat better reproducibility.

The ICS report also proposed an agar diffusion method that is a modification of that described in 1960 by Ericsson.[4] This procedure employs an inoculum that produces an almost confluent growth and that requires a 30-minute prediffusion period at room temperature before the plates are transferred to a 35°C incubator. In the United States, the Food and Drug Administration (FDA), acting upon the recommendation of an advisory committee, published the details of a standardized agar diffusion technique.[6,7] This method is a slight modification of the technique that Bauer et al. described in 1966.[3] It differs from the ICS method in that a slightly heavier inoculum is used and no prediffusion period is required. The National Committee for Clinical Laboratory Standards (NCCLS) also developed performance standards for antimicrobic disc susceptibility tests that outlined in greater detail the method published by the FDA. The agar overlay method of Barry et al. is recognized by both the NCCLS and the FDA as an acceptable alternative method for inoculation of the test plates.[2] The NCCLS document also outlines some general guidelines for selecting the microorganisms that ordinarily need susceptibility testing and for selecting the most relevant antimicrobial agents for routine testing. The NCCLS document contains guidelines for evaluating the performance of a clinical laboratory and the way in which the standard methods are actually utilized.[1]

Although these efforts have been directed primarily toward the development of standard reference methods, the techniques that have been described as national or international reference methods are perfectly suitable for routine use in clinical laboratories. In fact, the FDA and NCCLS documents specifically describe procedures that are practical for routine clinical laboratory use. These recommended techniques are outlined in the following chapters.

In summary, well-standardized techniques for antimicrobic susceptibility testing have been adequately described and tested on international and national levels. Use of techniques that deviate from these standard methods can be justified only after sufficient experimentation has clearly documented equal or superior accuracy and precision of the proposed modification. Most clinical laboratories do not have the space, time, personnel, nor expertise required to evaluate adequately modifications of the standard methods. In such laboratories, inappropriate deviation from the standard techniques is strongly discouraged. On the other hand, the standard reference methods can be used for evaluating innovations as they are developed by persons who have the capacity to undertake meaningful comparative studies.

SELECTION OF APPROPRIATE METHODS

What general type of test procedure is most appropriate for a given situation depends upon the equipment available, the number and type of microorganisms and antimicrobics to be studied, and the purpose for which the tests are being performed. Either agar diffusion or antimicrobic dilution tests may be used to:

1. Test individual isolates to provide a guide for selection of therapy.
2. Study the relative activity and antimicrobic spectrum of new agents.
3. Study microbial populations to document the shift in resistance patterns under selective effects of antimicrobic use.
4. Determine antibiograms as epidemiologic markers or for presumptive identification of an isolate.

In the clinical laboratory, most studies are performed for reasons Nos. 1 and 4, but other types of information can be collected by review of the laboratory's records. Generally, agar diffusion (disc) tests are adequate, but antimicrobic dilution techniques should be available to the clinical laboratory, particularly when special studies are to be undertaken. The agar diffusion test is the most convenient for day-to-day use and it is generally satisfactory when:

1. Simple qualitative information is sufficient.
2. The test strains are capable of growing at a fairly uniform rapid rate.
3. A fairly large number of drugs are to be studied at the same time.
4. Diffusion tests with the agents and microorganisms being tested have been standardized previously and shown to be satisfactory.

On the other hand, antimicrobic dilution tests may be required:

1. If more quantitative measures of susceptibility are needed.
2. If the test strains are relatively fastidious or slow growing.
3. If the number of drugs to be tested at one time can be limited to a practical number.
4. When diffusion tests have been found to be unsatisfactory for a particular agent or type of microorganism.
5. When the potential for lethal activity is to be determined.

Whether broth or agar dilution methods are to be selected depends upon a number of practical considerations. With an inoculum-replicating apparatus, the agar dilution method permits simultaneous testing of as many as 25 to 30 strains. The broth dilution method may be more convenient if only one or two strains are to be tested. If semi-automated microdilution techniques are used, individual strains can be tested conveniently against a fairly large number of agents at the one time. The agar dilution test has an advantage over the broth dilution method in that inhomogeneity of the inoculum can be detected readily. The inhomogeneity may be due to the presence of mixed cultures, to contamination, or to a resistant mutant in the inoculum. The broth dilution test provides only the MIC for the most resistant portion of the population within the inoculum. The broth dilution technique has two advantages over the agar dilution method: (1) the minimal lethal concentration (MLC) can be determined by subculturing an appropriate volume of the broth showing no growth, and (2) combinations of antimicrobics can be studied. Finally, agar dilution methods are more convenient for testing fastidious microorganisms that require the addition of blood or blood products to the test medium.

INDICATIONS FOR PERFORMING SUSCEPTIBILITY TESTS

Susceptibility tests that are performed to provide a guide for selection of the most appropriate therapeutic agent may be irrelevant if the test strain is not thoughtfully selected. Susceptibility tests are indicated for any microbial isolate that is thought to be contributing to an infectious process warranting chemotherapy, provided that its susceptibility or resistance cannot be predicted from a knowledge of its identity. When the nature of the infection is not clear and the specimen contains mixed growth or normal flora in which the microorganisms probably bear little relationship to the infectious process being treated, susceptibility tests are often wasteful and may be grossly misleading. Susceptibility tests are rarely necessary when the infection is due to a microorganism that is invariably susceptible to a highly effective drug. One example is the apparently universal susceptibility to penicillin among isolates of *Streptococcus pyogenes, S. pneumoniae,* and *Neisseria meningitidis.* On the other hand, susceptibility tests are most often indicated when the causative organism has been identified as a species known to be capable of exhibiting resistance to commonly used antimicrobial agents, especially *Staphylococcus* sp. and *Enterobacteriaceae.* Of course, that does not mean that a final identification must be accomplished before susceptibility tests are initiated.

It might be quite appropriate to test those isolates that ordinarily do not require susceptibility testing if one is attempting to study a new drug or to determine the overall incidence of resistance within a given population or to determine the antibiogram for epidemiologic purposes or to help in the presumptive identification of an isolate. However, the results of a test performed for these purposes should not be reported to the physician until the significance is explained to him.

In practice, isolated colonies of microorganisms that may be playing a pathogenic role should be selected from the primary agar plates and then tested under controlled conditions while the final identification procedures are being carried out. Mixtures of different types of microorganisms should never be tested in the same susceptibility test. The practice of inoculating susceptibility tests directly with clinical material should be reserved for the occasional clinical emergency. When such a procedure is performed, delayed indirect tests should always be carried out under better controlled conditions in order to confirm the preliminary results with the direct test.

Identification procedures should always be performed with separate single colony isolates since mixed cultures yield misleading biochemical and serological reactions. For susceptibility testing, the inoculum is traditionally derived from several colonies, and thus the possibility of obtaining mixed cultures in the inoculum is always present. Usually four or five well-isolated colonies of the same morphologic type are selected from the primary agar plate cultures. If stock cultures are being studied, they should be restreaked onto the appropriate agar medium and isolated colonies selected for testing after an adequate period of incubation; growth is never selected from stored slants or plates. The inoculum is prepared by transferring growth obtained by touching the top of each colony with an inoculating wire or loop to a tube containing an appropriate broth medium. Sampling several colonies is thought to reduce the chance of selecting a variant derived from loss-mutation, such as loss of penicillinase production of *Staphylococcus aureus* or segregants from R factor resistance markers. It also increases the chance of including representatives of a more resistant variant that may be present but cannot be distinguished morphologically from the more susceptible variants within the same population. Admittedly, the selection of four or five colonies from thousands of colonies does not represent a statistically valid sample; it is a practical compromise with reality, certainly more representative of the predominant components than is a single colony isolate.

REFERENCES

1. Barry, A. L. 1974. The role of NCCLS in standardization of antimicrobic susceptibility techniques. In *Current Techniques for Antibiotic Susceptibility Testing*. A. Balows (Ed.). Charles C Thomas, Springfield, Ill. pp. 47-53.
2. Barry, A. L., F. Garcia, and L. D. Thrupp. 1970. An improved method for testing the antibiotic susceptibility of rapidly growing pathogens. Am. J. Clin. Pathol. 53: 149-158.
3. Bauer, A. W., W. M. M. Kirby, J. C. Sherris, and M. Turck. 1966. Antibiotic susceptibility testing by a standardized single disk method. Am. J. Clin. Pathol. 45: 493-496.
4. Ericsson, H. 1960. The paper disc method for determination of bacterial sensitivity to antibiotics. J. Clin. & Lab. Invest. 12: 1-15.

5. Ericsson, H. M., and J. C. Sherris. 1971. Antibiotic sensitivity testing. Report of an international collaborative study. Acta Pathol. Microbiol. Scand. Sect. B, Suppl. 217.
6. Federal Register. 1972. Rules and regulations. Antibiotic susceptibility discs. Fed. Regist. *37:* 20525-20529.
7. Federal Register. 1973. Rules and regulations. Antibiotic susceptibility discs: Correction. Fed. Regist. *38:* 2576.
8. Fleming, A. 1929. On the antibacterial action of cultures of a penicillium, with special reference to their use in the isolation of *B. influenzae*. Br. J. Exp. Pathol. *10:* 226-236.
9. Florey, H. W., E. Chain, N. G. Heatley, and M. E. Florey. 1949. *Antibiotics.* 1st ed. Oxford Univ. Press, London.
10. Hoeprich, P. D. 1971. In search of a word. J. Infect. Dis. *123:* 225.
11. Schoenknecht, F. D., and J. C. Sherris. 1972. New perspectives in antibiotic susceptibility testing. In *Recent Advances in Clinical Pathology.* S. C. Dyke (Ed.). Churchill Livingstone, Edinburgh. pp. 272-292.
12. World Health Organization. 1961. Standardization of methods for conducting microbic sensitivity tests. *Second Report of the Expert Committee on Antibiotics.* World Health Organization Technical Reports Series No. 210, pp. 1-24.
13. Wright, W. W. 1974. FDA actions on antibiotic susceptibility discs. In *Current Techniques for Antibiotic Susceptibility Testing.* A. Balows (Ed.). Charles C Thomas, Springfield, Ill. pp. 26-46.

Chapter **2**

DEFINITION OF TERMS "RESISTANT" AND "SUSCEPTIBLE"

Definition of the terms "resistant" and "susceptible" is fundamental to any discussion of antimicrobial susceptibility tests. These terms are often used to describe slightly different phenomena and deserve further qualification. From a strict biologic point of view, the terms "resistant" and "susceptible" may be used to express the ability or lack of ability of a microorganism to multiply in the presence of a given concentration of antimicrobic under defined conditions. Within a single bacterial population, some individual cells may be resistant to a certain concentration of antimicrobic, whereas other individual cells might be susceptible to that concentration. In the same sense, an individual strain may be said to be susceptible to a given concentration of antimicrobic if a large majority of individual cells within the culture are inhibited by that concentration, whereas another strain may be said to be resistant to that concentration of antimicrobic if it is capable of growing under defined test conditions. In practice, the degree of susceptibility is often expressed quantitatively as the lowest concentration of drug that inhibits the growth of a given strain. This is normally expressed as the minimal inhibitory concentration (MIC), the minimal concentration of antimicrobic that results in complete or nearly complete inhibition of growth under specified test conditions. Since MIC values are generally determined by inoculating a series of doubling dilutions of the antimicrobic, a strain is resistant to a concentration equal to one-half the MIC. In reality, the "true" MIC falls somewhere between the expressed MIC and 50% of that value and is influenced by a number of technologic variables that can influence the end-point rather dramatically.

From a clinician's point of view, a microorganism may be considered "susceptible" to a particular antimicrobial agent if *in vitro* studies suggest that a patient infected by that microorganism is likely to respond favorably to the drug when it is given in dosages appropriate to the type of microorganism and the type of infection. The term "resistant" then implies that the infection is not likely to respond to such therapy (i.e., the MIC exceeds the concentration of drug that can be expected at the site of infection).

Such a simplistic definition cannot be applied realistically without considering a number of complicating variables that must be taken into account before attempting to predict the response of an individual patient to chemotherapy with a specific drug or combination of drugs. The terms "resistant" and "susceptible" are probably best thought of as arbitrary categories designating the extremes of a spectrum joined by an intermediate category that nearly defies unqualified definition. With those microorganisms that fall at the extremes that may be confidently labeled susceptible or resistant, therapeutic responsiveness or unresponsiveness may be reasonably anticipated. A number of host factors influence the final outcome. The factors cannot be measured by an *in vitro* test system but they must be taken into account when interpreting the results of the *in vitro* tests.

HOST FACTORS INFLUENCING THE OUTCOME OF ANTIMICROBIC CHEMOTHERAPY

In general, antimicrobics function by inhibiting microbial growth long enough to permit the host to remove the invading microorganisms from the site of infection. If, for some reason, the patient's defense mechanisms are not functioning optimally, the infection might not be influenced by chemotherapy, or, at best, it might initially appear to respond, only to recur once the drug is discontinued. In such situations, prolonged chemotherapy will eventually encourage the selection of resistant variants or invite a secondary infection with a more resistant strain. If the host's cellular or immunologic defense mechanisms are compromised by pathologic or iatrogenic means, infections due to fully susceptible microorganisms may not respond satisfactorily. For example, normally satisfactory chemotherapy may not be adequate in the patient with acute leukemia or uncontrolled diabetes mellitus under treatment with supraphysiologic doses of glucosteroids or in patients receiving other suppressants of immune response. For the same reasons, infections localized at sites protected from the phagocytic system might also fail to respond completely. For example, when the invading microorganism is lodged within an abscess or within the vegetation of an endocarditis, the phagocytic system is not capable of operating optimally, although the antimicrobic penetrates to the site of infection. Incision and drainage of abscesses are essential to the success of antimicrobial chemotherapy. When this procedure is not possible, such therapy will be of limited value even though the microorganism is fully susceptible to the antimicrobic in use. In such situations, a bactericidal drug, or combination of drugs, might be advantageous if it is capable of reaching the site of infection in sufficient concentration.

On the other hand, microorganisms resistant to concentrations ordinarily obtained in the blood might respond to therapy if the infection is located in an organ system in which the drug is normally concentrated, e.g., the urinary tract.

The natural course of the type of infection being treated should also be considered. Infections that normally carry a high morbidity and mortality are often treated more intensely than infections that are less serious. Chemotherapy of the less serious infections is often difficult to evaluate since the patient may appear to respond to the antimicrobial agent given at the time the infection would be eliminated naturally. Apparent success in treating an infection due to microorganisms properly classified as resistant may be quite common with such a self-limiting disease. At the other extreme, patients with serious underlying disease might fail to survive although their infection was appropriately treated with an antimicrobic to which the etiologic agent was susceptible *in vitro*.

In summary, the efficacy of a particular antimicrobial agent depends upon a number of factors, among them:

1. Degree of susceptibility of the invading microorganism
2. Concentration of drug obtained at the site of the infection (dosage, or biological and pharmacological properties of the particular drug preparation being used)
3. Location of the infection
4. Pathophysiologic state of the patient
5. Natural history of the infection

6. Nature and severity of the infection
7. Application of other supportive therapeutic measures, e.g., prompt incision and drainage of abscesses.

Once the presence of an infection is established and the etiologic agent identified, the physician must decide whether chemotherapy is needed. If it is, he must select the most appropriate agent for the particular patient. All the above-mentioned factors must be considered systematically in selecting the most appropriate course of therapy for each particular patient. The susceptibility of the microorganism may be determined *in vitro* with various types of susceptibility tests. The concentration of drug at the site of infection may be determined for each individual patient by directly assaying the antimicrobic in the body fluids; however, it is usually estimated from a knowledge of the pharmacokinetics of the particular drug and preparation being considered. To determine the final course of action, such *in vitro* determinations provide important information that must be meshed with knowledge of other factors that cannot be measured in the laboratory.

CATEGORIZATION OF SUSCEPTIBILITY

Although *in vitro* susceptibility is only one of many factors that determine the final effect of chemotherapy, it is possible to develop interpretive guidelines that help predict whether most infections will be responsive or nonresponsive to therapy. This can be done only by using those criteria that can be measured in a rather artificial *in vitro* environment. Based on such *in vitro* data, microorganisms may be categorized into susceptible or resistant groups, with one or more intermediate categories between these two extremes. Two distinctly different definitions of the qualitative terms "susceptible" and "resistant" must be considered.

Definition 1. A microorganism is susceptible if it is inhibited by a concentration of antimicrobic that is less than that normally obtained in the blood of patients treated with doses of the drug that are normally given for the type of infection and type of microorganism in question.

Conversely, a microorganism is considered resistant if inhibition occurs only with concentrations well above those normally obtained in the blood during such therapy. Between these two groups, there may be an intermediate category consisting of a relatively small group of microorganisms inhibited by concentrations equal to or slightly higher than that normally obtained in the blood during therapy with the usual dosage. Those strains with intermediate susceptibility might respond to treatment if dose and route of administration are adjusted to obtain greater than normal concentrations of the antimicrobic at the site of infection.

Such a working definition is based on the common assumption that the concentration of antimicrobic in the blood serves as a practical guide for predicting the concentration in various tissues. Blood is the most readily available tissue for assay, and is actually the transport medium that delivers the drug to the site of the infection. In practice, tissue concentrations are usually assumed to be somewhat lower than the maximal concentration achieved in the blood. In fact, there are few studies actually documenting the concentration of the drug at different sites of the body. The passage of an antimicrobial agent into various tissues, secretions, and compartments of the body is favored by: (1) increased concentration in the blood, (2) small molecular size, (3) absence of an electrical charge at a physiologic pH, (4) solubility in lipids, and (5) absence of binding (or loose binding) to plasma proteins. Consequently, no broad generalization can be made concerning the ratio between blood levels and the concentrations in various tissues since it will vary with the tissue and the agent under consideration. In spite of this, the blood remains the most useful tissue for assaying the concentration achieved in the body.

The "average blood level" is somewhat of a misnomer since the actual concentration in the blood varies in different persons given the same dosage, especially if the dosage is not carefully adjusted according to the total body mass. Even then, individuals vary somewhat in their capacity to absorb the drug from the site of administration (especially when the drug is given orally), to eliminate the drug, as in the urine or bile, or to catabolize the drug in the liver, kidneys, or other organs. This is particularly true in patients with abnormal function of those organs responsible for excretion or catabolism of the drug.

When the drug is given by continuous intravenous administration, the dosage may be adjusted to reach a fairly steady state at the desired concentration. However, intermittent injection by intravenous or intramuscular routes or by oral administration results in a rather remarkable fluctuation in blood levels at various times between doses. The transient peak concentration is often much greater than the lowest concentration, which occurs just before the next dose. "Average peak blood level" is a term often used to express the usual concentration in the average patient at a time when the peak level is anticipated. The "mean blood level" may be defined as the mid-point value between the highest and lowest concentration obtained during intermittent therapy.

In spite of these disadvantages and uncertainties, the approximate concentration of drug expected in the blood of a patient is a useful criterion in predicting the susceptibility or resistance of a given microorganism. The approximate range of peak blood levels frequently obtained with some commonly used antimicrobial agents is shown in Table 2-1. As a guideline, one may consider an

Table 2-1. Peak Serum Concentrations Frequently Obtained with Some Antimicrobial Agents

Antimicrobial Agent	Serum Conc. (μg/ml)
Penicillins†	
Depot (benzathine penicillin G)	0.01–0.06
Depot (procaine penicillin G)	0.1–18
Oral	3–20‡
Intramuscular or intravenous	2–200‡
Cephalothin	15–150
Cephaloridine	14–28
Cefazolin	38–118
Cephalexin	5–35
Tetracycline	
Oral	1–5
Intravenous	5–30
Doxycycline	1–6
Minocycline	0.7–4.5
Clindamycin	5–26
Lincomycin	2–20
Erythromycin	2–10
Gentamicin	1–8
Kanamycin	10–25
Streptomycin	10–25
Chloramphenicol	3–12
Vancomycin	20–50
Polymyxin B	2–8
Colistin	6
Sulfonamides	100–150
Isoniazid	2–3
Rifampin	10
Ethambutol	5–10
Metronidazol	4–10
Amphotericin B	0.2–2
5-Fluorocytosine	20–100

Source: L. D. Sabath. 1974. In *Manual of Clinical Microbiology*, 2d ed. E. H. Lennette, E. H. Spaulding, and J. P. Truant (Eds.). American Society for Microbiology, Washington, D. C. p. 442.

† Penicillins include benzylpenicillin, phenoxymethylpenicillin, ampicillin, amoxicillin, carbenicillin, methicillin, oxacillin, cloxacillin, dicloxacillin, and nafcillin.

‡ Wide ranges represent the effect of different doses, routes of administration, and/or preparations.

organism to be susceptible if it is inhibited by a concentration at least one-half the mean blood level or one-fourth the average peak blood level, whereas it is considered to be resistant if the MIC is greater than the peak blood level. The imprecision of such generalizations must be appreciated in order to understand the difficulty in defining "resistance" and "susceptibility" in exact terms.

Therapy of urinary tract infections deserves special mention because some investigators feel that a different set of criteria should be developed. Many antimicrobics are excreted through the kidneys and are concentrated in the urine in levels much greater than those obtained in the blood. Some microorganisms that are resistant to an antimicrobic at concentrations found in the blood stream are susceptible to concentrations found in the urine. Urinary tract infections caused by such microorganisms may respond to therapy if the site of infection is located in an area exposed to the urine. When the urinary tract infection is localized at a site not directly confluent with the urine (e.g., perinephric abscess), blood levels are likely to be more relevant guides. In either case, antimicrobics that are effective at concentrations obtained in the blood should be effective in treating urinary tract infections. However, although the microorganism is resistant to ordinary blood levels, less expensive and less toxic drugs might be equally effective if higher concentrations result from urinary excretion.

Within the limits of precision inherent in the method used, the MIC value can be related to approximate concentrations expected at the site of infection in order to predict responsiveness or nonresponsiveness to treatment of the infected patient. Another approach to interpretation is based upon identification of two distinct populations within strains belonging to the same species. A second definition emphasizes the relative value of one MIC determination as compared to others done in the same way.

Definition 2. An individual strain may be considered resistant if it tolerates a concentration of antimicrobic appreciably higher than one that inhibits growth of the majority of other strains within that species.

In this sense of the word, "resistance" is a relative term meaning "less susceptible than that usually encountered" and by itself does not necessarily suggest nonresponsiveness to chemotherapy. With many antimicrobial agents, different strains within a species show an unimodal distribution of MICs spread over a narrow range. When the MICs are well below the anticipated blood levels, the species may be said to be uniformally susceptible—provided that practical experience confirms clinical responsiveness to chemotherapy. With selective pressures resulting from widespread chemotherapeutic use of the drug, resistant mutants or recombinants may appear within a population. This can result in a clear-cut bimodal distribution of strains, one population being much more resistant than the other. If the MIC values for the more resistant population exceed the anticipated blood level and if clinical experience suggests such strains might not be expected to respond to chemotherapy, then they may be correctly labeled as resistant in every sense of the word. For this reason, knowledge of the behavior of an individual strain in relationship to others within the same species may be of considerable predictive value. For comparative purposes, the approximate MIC values usually observed with susceptible strains of some of the more common bacterial pathogens are listed in Table 2-2. Because of variability between strains and differences in methodology, the actual MIC may vary two or three doubling dilutions above or below the mode. Strains showing appreciably greater MICs might be considered members of a "resistant" population, i.e., less susceptible than the normal population, provided that susceptible control strains were tested at the same time and produced MIC's within the expected range for the susceptible population.

The practical value of this approach is exemplified by the data in Figure 2-1. The results of agar dilution tests are summarized to give

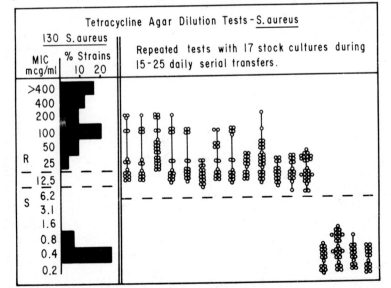

Figure 2-1. Reproducibility of tetracycline MICs with resistant and susceptible strains of *S. aureus*. (Adapted from A. L. Barry, 1962. Ph.D. diss. Ohio State University.)

Table 2-2. Approximate MICs (μg/ml) Expected with the More Susceptible Strains among Some Common Bacterial Pathogens (excluding Resistant Variants and Recombinants)

Organism	Erythromycin	Clindamycin	Nafcillin	Benzylpenicillin	Ampicillin	Carbenicillin	Cephalothin	Tetracycline	Chloramphenicol	Polymyxin B (units/ml)	Streptomycin	Kanamycin	Gentamicin	Nitrofurantoin	Nalidixic acid
S. aureus Penicillinase negative	0.25	0.06	0.5	0.06	0.12	1.0	0.8	0.5	8.0	>128	4.0	2.0	0.5	16	>128
Streptococcus sp. α- or nonhemolytic	0.01	0.01	0.12	0.12	0.12	2.0	0.25	0.5	2.0	>128	8.0	64	4.0		
Enterococci	0.40	16	16	4.0	2.0	64	16	1.0	8.0	>128	128	64	8.0	32	>128
Escherichia	128	>128	>128	64	4.0	4.0	8.0	8.0	8.0	4.0	4.0	4.0	1.0	16	4.0
Klebsiella	>128	>128	>128	>128	64	>128	4.0	4.0	4.0	4.0	4.0	4.0	0.5	128	8.0
Enterobacter	>128	>128	>128	>128	>128	4.0	>128	4.0	8.0	8.0	4.0	4.0	1.0	64	4.0
Serratia	>128	>128	>128	>128	128	>128	>128	>128	16	>128	4.0		1.0	256	
Proteus P. mirabilis	>128	>128	>128	8.0	2.0	2.0	4.0	64	16	>128	8.0	4.0	1.0	128	8.0
Other species	>128	>128	>128	>128	32	2.0	>128	64	8.0	>128	4.0	2.0	0.5	64	8.0
P. aeruginosa	>128	>128	>128	>128	>128	64	>128	64	>128	16	64	128	2.0	>256	>256
H. influenzae	4.0	4.0	>128	0.5	0.5	0.5	16	1.0	1.0	>128	4.0	2.0	0.5	>256	
B. fragilis	2.0	0.5	>128	16	16	32	64	1.0	8.0	>128	>128	>128	>128	>128	>128

SOURCE: A. L. Barry. 1974. In *Manual of Clinical Microbiology*, 2d ed. E. H. Lennette, E. H. Spaulding, and J. P. Truant (Eds.). American Society for Microbiology, Washington D. C. p. 441.)

NOTE: The values listed represent an estimate of the modal MIC when a fairly large series of strains is tested. In most cases, the MIC for a normal member of the population can be expected to fall within two dilutions above or below the mode. In different studies, the mode may differ among strains because of differences in methodology. The above data were based largely upon broth and agar dilution studies (A. L. Barry. Unpublished data) supplemented with data collected from a large variety of published works in which similar methods were used.

a profile of resistance to tetracycline among isolates of *Staphylococcus aureus*. Initial tests with 130 isolates demonstrated a clear-cut bimodal distribution of MICs, one population being well above and the other being well below the usual blood level. Seventeen strains were selected eight months later from the original 130 stock cultures, and tests were repeated daily for from 15 to 25 consecutive days. Upon continual retesting of strains within the susceptible population, individual MIC determinations varied no more than one doubling dilution above or below the mode. However, with strains drawn from the resistant population, the MIC values were more variable. Although an individual determination for a given strain may vary within the limits prescribed for that population, susceptible strains are readily distinguished from those belonging to the resistant population. Upon repeated testing, the resistant strains occasionally gave MICs within the upper limits of obtainable blood levels, but at other times each strain gave MICs greater than the anticipated blood levels. If a single MIC determination were made and strictly interpreted according to the criterion set down in Definition 1 (p. 15), the interpretation of tests with susceptible strains would not vary from day to day; however, some resistant strains would be considered moderately susceptible or resistant on different days. On the other hand, if the bimodal distribution of MICs were considered and the MIC break points between resistant and susceptible shifted downward slightly, the interpretation of the tests would not be altered. In addition to reducing the impact of the technical variability inherent in the dilution procedure, such an adjustment of MIC breakpoints would partially compensate for the apparent disparity between blood and tissue concentrations.

With other genera, clear-cut bimodal distribution of MIC values is less readily identified. Table 2-3 demonstrates results of similar agar dilution tests with *Staphylococcus aureus* and with five commonly encountered gram-negative genera. The susceptible enteric bacilli are from 5 to 10 times less susceptible than *S. aureus*. With most gram-negative genera, some strains display MICs so close to the arbitrary breakpoints that occasional errors of interpretation result (assuming that there is some degree of variability within the population). Careful standardization and quality control of the dilution technique is especially important with such microorganisms.

Table 2-4 summarizes the same type of data with another drug, cephalothin. In this particular series of tests, the *Klebsiella* sp. and the *Proteus* sp. generally gave a range of MICs below obtainable blood levels. The *Enterobacter* sp. and *Pseudomonas aeruginosa*

Table 2-3. Tetracycline Agar Dilution MICs with Six Commonly Encountered Bacterial Pathogens

Genus	Number of Tests	1.0	2.5	5	10	25	50	>50
Staphylococcus	130	31*				3	9	57
Escherichia	115	2	44	36		2	2	14
Klebsiella	72	1	30	42	14	5		8
Enterobacter	53		9	68	4		1	18
Proteus	34				1	1	84	14
Pseudomonas	52						23	6

SOURCE: A. L. Barry and L. D. Thrupp. Unpublished data.
* Percent inhibited: inoculum approximately 3×10^5 cells per plate.

Table 2-4. Cephalothin Agar Dilution MICs with Five Commonly Encountered Gram-Negative Bacilli

Genus	Number of Tests	2.5	5	10	25	50	100	>100
Escherichia	119	4*	10	23	41	14	4	4
Klebsiella	106	5	52	26	10	4	1	2
Enterobacter	53						2	98
Proteus	76	4	51	30	12			3
Pseudomonas	55							100

SOURCE: A. L. Barry and L. D. Thrupp. Unpublished data.
* Percent inhibited: inoculum approximately 3×10^5 cells per plate.

were both resistant. With *Escherichia coli*, the MICs were broadly distributed, and the mode fell into the intermediate category. A modification of the method for determining MIC values, e.g., reduction in inoculum size, would easily shift the MIC values so that a large proportion would fall into the susceptible category (Fig. 2-2). Alternatively, the interpretive breakpoints for testing with a heavy inoculum could be shifted upward by one doubling dilution. Either maneuver would cause most *E. coli* to appear to be susceptible and would not significantly influence the interpretation of tests with the other gram-negative bacilli. Such manipulations of testing methods or of blood level–based breakpoints is justifiable only if clinical experience in treating infections caused by *E. coli* with cephalothin results in a favorable outcome and therefore supports an interpretation of susceptible.

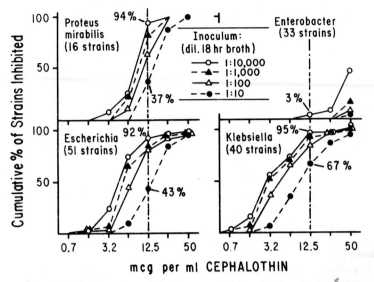

Figure 2-2. Distribution of cephalothin agar dilution MICs with four different inoculum densities. (From A. L. Barry, and L. D. Thrupp. Unpublished data.)

Nitrofurantoin cannot be detected in the blood, but high concentrations are found in the urine. Consequently, interpretations of MICs must be based on urine rather than blood levels. Although urinary concentrations as high as 500 μg/ml or more may be reached, concentrations of at least 50 μg/ml are usually maintained for several hours after oral administration of the drug. Clinically, most strains with MICs of 50 μg/ml or less generally respond to therapy,whereas those strains with MICs of 250 μg/ml or more rarely respond. Those strains with MICs between these extremes are best considered intermediate in susceptibility. The distribution of nitrofurantoin MIC values with five genera is summarized in Table 2-5. Each of the genera yielded a fairly well defined unimodal distribution of values: the *E. coli* were clearly susceptible and the *Pseudomonas aeruginosa* definitely resistant. Both the *Klebsiella* sp. and the *Enterobacter* sp. gave MIC values broadly distributed on either side of the mode. These represent a group of microorganisms that are neither susceptible nor resistant and are best classified as having intermediate susceptibility; they may respond to treatment with nitrofurantoin if high concentrations can be maintained at the site of infection for a sufficiently long period. The percentage of *Klebsiella* sp. or *Enterobacter* sp. inhibited by 50 μg/ml is influenced markedly by the *in vitro* test conditions, especially the density of the inoculum (Fig. 2-3). The interpretation of

Table 2-5. Nitrofurantoin Agar Dilution MICs with Five
Commonly Encountered Gram-Negative Bacilli

Genus	Number of Tests	μg/ml Nitrofurantoin					
		10	25	50	100	250	≥500
Escherichia	105	7*	92	1			
Klebsiella	100		6	17	37	36	4
Enterobacter	51			11	57	27	5
Proteus	61				20	80	
Pseudomonas	52					1	99

SOURCE: Data from A. L. Barry and L. D. Thrupp. 1968. Antimicrob. Agents Chemother. *8:*418.

* Percent inhibited: inoculum approximately 3 × 10⁵ cells per plate.

tests with *Escherichia coli* or *Proteus* sp. is not influenced greatly by variations in the inoculum.

Estimates of the mean and the peak blood levels are based on observations made during chemotherapy with the usual dosage for a particular type of infection and type of microorganism. The "usual dosage" varies somewhat with regional or individual practices. Different dosage schedules are often recommended for different sites of infection and for different types of microorganisms. Con-

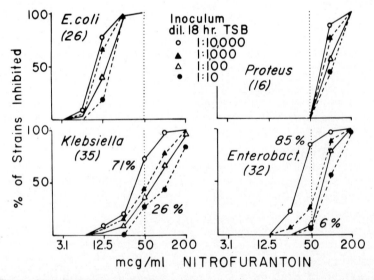

Figure 2-3. Distribution of nitrofurantoin agar dilution MICs with four different inoculum densities. (From A. L. Barry, and L. D. Thrupp. 1969. Antimicrob. Agents Chemother. *8:*420.)

sequently, it may be necessary to describe separate interpretative criteria for different situations. For example, with carbenicillin, the dosage recommended for treating infections caused by *Pseudomonas aeruginosa* exceeds that suggested for treating infections caused by *Escherichia coli* or *Proteus* sp. Thus, two types of interpretative criteria are described, depending upon the species being tested. It would be equally logical to establish dual standards for interpreting tests with other drugs for which dosage schedules may vary according to the kind of microorganism and/or organ system involved.

It should be obvious that no single set of interpretative criteria can be applied blindly to all clinical situations. A system that simply separates the susceptible and resistant categories is often inadequate. With many drugs, a third, intermediate, category is necessary in order to identify those strains that are clearly neither resistant nor susceptible. In spite of these difficulties, some type of system for categorization of susceptibility is necessary in order to interpret *in vitro* susceptibility tests.

In response to such problems, a working committee of the International Collaborative Study recommended Ericsson's four-category system, which takes into consideration differences in dosage schedules. Because of difficulties that would be encountered in translating descriptive terms into different languages, the categories were simply labeled Groups 1 through 4. These four groups may be defined as follows:

Group 1 (very susceptible) includes strains with such high degrees of susceptibility that *in vivo* response is probable when mild-to-moderately-severe systemic infections are treated with the usual dosage of antimicrobic, given orally when applicable.

Group 2 (fairly susceptible) includes strains with degrees of susceptibility that make *in vivo* response probable in patients with systemic infections when the antimicrobic is given in high dosage or up to the limits of toxicity.

Group 3 (moderately resistant) includes strains with degrees of susceptibility that make *in vivo* response probable only when treating infections localized at sites where the agent will be concentrated by physiologic processes or by local application.

Group 4 (resistant) includes strains with degrees of resistance that makes *in vivo* response improbable.

Wherever possible, to give each group statistical validity, the differences between groups should be at least three doubling dilution steps. Not all groups need to be used for each antimicrobic. For example, with the polymyxins, no Group 1 designation is allocated (and thus these drugs should not be considered first-line antimicrobics) and no Group 3 designation is allocated (because of the potential for toxicity).

One such set of guidelines for interpretation is presented in Table 2-6.

Although such a four-category system has many advantages, it has not been widely accepted in the United States, where a two- or three-category system is generally preferred and where Groups 3 and 4 are often considered resistant and Groups 1 and 2 susceptible. With some drugs, a third, intermediate, category is often designated to describe those strains that are neither clearly resistant nor clearly susceptible. Regardless of whether two, three, or four

Table 2-6. Suggested Guidelines for Interpretation of Antimicrobic Dilution Test Results: Four-Category System

Antimicrobial Agent	Range of MICs (μg/ml) Each Category*			
	Very Susceptible	Fairly Susceptible	Moderately Resistant	Very Resistant
Penicillin	≤0.125†	0.25– 8.0	16–128	> 128
Ampicillin	≤ 0.25†	0.5– 8.0	16–128	> 128
Carbenicillin	≤ 32	64–256	X‡	> 256
Methicillin	≤ 4.0	X	X	> 4
Oxacillin	≤ 2.0	X	X	> 2
Cephalothin	≤ 2.0	4.0– 16	32–128	> 128
Kanamycin	≤ 2.0	4.0– 8.0	16–64	> 64
Gentamicin	≤ 0.5	1.0– 4.0	8–64	> 64
Chloramphenicol	≤ 1.0	2.0– 8.0	X	≥ 16
Tetracycline	≤ 1.0	2.0– 8.0	16–32	> 32
Erythromycin	≤ 1.0	2.0– 4.0	8.0–16	> 16
Clindamycin	≤ 1.0	2.0– 4.0	8.0–16	> 16
Polymyxins§	X	≤2.0	X	≥ 4.0
Sulfonamides	≤ 20	40– 80	160–1280	>1280
Nitrofurantoin‖	≤ 32	64–128	X	≥ 256

* See text for further definition of the four categories.

† When testing *S. aureus*, MICs of 0.5 μg/ml or more should be considered evidence of penicillinase production and thus interpreted as being very resistant.

‡ Classification of bacteria into categories thus marked is considered inappropriate for that particular drug.

§ Includes polymyxin B or E (colistin sulfate or colistin methane-sulfonate), expressed as μg/ml.

‖ Results apply only to urinary tract infections since detectable blood levels of nitrofurantoin are not obtained during therapy.

categories are designated, selection of the breakpoints is based largely upon three general types of information, which can be summarized as follows:

1. The amount of drug expected at the site of infection is related to the concentration required for *in vitro* inhibition of growth (the MIC). It is recognized that even under the best of standardized conditions the MIC determination itself has some degree of inherent variability. Furthermore, if the *in vitro* test conditions are altered, the actual MIC value may be shifted rather dramatically. Such an estimate of *in vitro* susceptibility is then related to the concentration of drug anticipated at the site of infection, as reflected by the peak or mean blood level expected with the usual dosage schedule. A number of variables influence the actual concentration obtained at the site of infection, and thus the concentration obtained *in vivo* cannot be defined in exacting terms. Because of the uncertainties inherent in this type of relationship, some kind of safety factor is often added to the equation, e.g., an organism may be considered susceptible if its MIC is at least one-half or one-fourth the anticipated mean blood level.

2. The overall distribution of MIC values with relevant clinical isolates should be examined. Breakpoints might be shifted slightly to avoid passing through the center of a distinct unimodal population and to minimize the number of strains that would fall into the intermediate category. Where a distinct bimodal distribution of MICs can be identified, the breakpoints should pass between the two populations.

3. Previous clinical experience with the therapy of infection due to different genera is taken into account in adjusting the MIC breakpoint in order to best reflect the most likely response.

From the above discussion it is clear that such a categorization scheme involves some degree of subjectivity and best-judgment decisions. For that reason, selection of breakpoints to be used in any standardized procedure should be made by a broadly based panel, one made up of experts in infectious diseases, microbiology, and the pharmacology of chemotherapeutics. Furthermore, the categories should be reviewed and updated periodically as further experience and knowledge accumulate.

EXCEPTIONS TO THE RULE

In testing strains of *Staphylococcus aureus* there are two situations in which quantitative susceptibility tests are not subject to the type of interpretation discussed above. These exceptions involve tests with benzylpenicillin and with the methicillin family of drugs. In both cases, clinical isolates that deviate from the susceptible population are best considered resistant, regardless of MIC values.

With benzylpenicillin, susceptible strains of *S. aureus* are generally inhibited by 0.05 μg/ml (± 1 doubling dilution), whereas those strains that require more than 0.1 μg/ml for inhibition are best considered resistant because they are capable of producing a penicillin-inactivating enzyme—penicillinase. The MIC value obtained with penicillinase-producing strains of *S. aureus* is particularly dependent upon testing conditions, especially on the inoculum size. For example, the very same strain may display MIC values ranging from 0.5 µg/ml to over 100 µg/ml under different test conditions. Clinical isolates that demonstrate resistance by mechanisms other than penicillinase production have not been encountered. A direct test for the capacity to produce penicillinase would be more meaningful to the clinician than a quantitative susceptibility test (Chapter 9). Methicillin, nafcillin and isoxazolyl penicillins (oxacillin, cloxacillin, dicloxacillin, flucloxacillin) are relatively resistant to the activity of penicillinase. Thus they are effective against penicillin-resistant staphylococci. However, some strains of *S. aureus* are resistant to the penicillinase-resistant penicillins by other mechanisms. Such resistant strains are heterogenous, i.e., the majority of cells in a particular clone may be fully susceptible but a small proportion have variable but definite resistance. The resistant portion of the population may not be detected on the usual isotonic medium incubated at 37°C, especially if a small inoculum is used. Susceptible strains are normally inhibited by 4 µg of methicillin per ml or 2 µg of nafcillin or oxacillin per ml, whereas resistant strains require much greater concentrations for inhibition. The actual MIC determination for resistant strains depends very much on the test conditions. Thus it is difficult, if not impossible, to relate MICs to blood levels.

In these two exceptional cases, a simple, qualitative distinction between resistant and susceptible strains is most appropriate and the method of choice is the one that provides a clear distinction between the two populations.

REFERENCES

1. Barry, A. L. 1963. The development of methods for determining antibiotic susceptibility. Am. J. Med. Technol. *29:* 298-304.
2. Bauer, A. W. 1964. The two definitions of bacterial resistance. In *Proceedings of the Third International Congress of Chemotherapy*. Stuttgart, Germany. pp. 484-500.
3. Branch, A., D. H. Starkey, and E. A. Power. 1965. Diversification in the tube dilution test for antibiotic sensitivity of microorganisms. Appl. Microbiol. *13:* 469-472.
4. Ericsson, H. M., and J. C. Sherris. 1971. Antibiotic sensitivity testing. Report of an international collaborative study. Acta Pathol. Microbiol. Scand. Sect. B, Suppl. 217.
5. Garrod, L. P., H. P. Lambert, and F. O'Grady (with a chapter on laboratory methods by P. M. Waterworth). 1973. *Antibiotic and Chemotherapy*. 4th ed. Churchill Livingstone, Edinburgh.
6. Goodman, L. S., and A. Gilman. 1970. *The Pharmacological Basis of Therapeutics*. 4th ed. Macmillan, New York.
7. Hoeprich, P. D. 1972. Antimicrobics and antihelmintics for systemic therapy. In *Infectious Diseases*. P. D. Hoeprich (Ed.). Harper & Row, Hagerstown, Maryland. pp. 177-206.

8. Lorian, V. 1966. *Antibiotics and Chemotherapeutic Agents in Clinical and Laboratory Practice.* Charles C Thomas, Springfield, Ill.
9. The Medical Letter on Drugs and Therapeutics. 1974. *Handbook of Antimicrobial Therapy.* The Medical Letter, Inc., New Rochelle, N. Y.
10. Schoenknecht, F. D., and J. C. Sherris. 1972. New perspectives in antibiotic susceptibility testing. In *Recent Advances in Clinical Pathology.* S. C. Dyke (Ed.). Churchill Livingstone, Edinburgh. pp. 272-292.
11. Thrupp, L. D. 1974. Significance and interpretation of quantitative antimicrobial susceptibility testing in clinical microbiology. In *Current Techniques for Antibiotic Susceptibility Testing.* A. Balows (Ed.). Charles C Thomas, Springfield, Ill. pp. 94-108.

Chapter 3

AN OVERVIEW OF ANTIMICROBICS

Paul D. Hoeprich, M.D.

As the number of antimicrobial agents burgeoned, a scheme of classification became necessary. Naturally at first, reference to the origins of drugs appeared to be sufficient. However, classification of antimicrobics according to origin became unsatisfactory when semi-synthesis yielded compounds valuable to therapy, e.g., the semi-synthetic penicillins.

An alternative classification referred to the kinds of microorganisms affected. It was an approach initially of general informing value, but grew less useful as more antimicrobics were introduced. However, if the limits of two definitions are heeded, some utility remains: *broad spectrum* refers to agents that are active against more than one of the major varieties of microorganisms, e.g., tetracyclines against chlamydias, rickettsias, mycoplasmas, and bacteria; *narrow spectrum* denotes agents that affect only one variety of microorganism, e.g., penicillins against bacteria.

The mechanisms of action of all antimicrobics are not known, and some agents act by more than one mechanism. Hence, classification cannot depend on mechanisms of action.

Because the chemical structure of an antimicrobic is an immutable characteristic of that drug, it remains the most generally applicable and unequivocal basis for classification. The antimicrobics to be discussed in this chapter are listed by chemical structure in Table 3-1, in the order in which they are reviewed.

AMINOCYCLITOLS

Of the aminocyclitols now on the market, those of current major interest for systemic therapy include streptomycin, kanamycin, gentamicin, and spectinomycin (used only for the treatment of gonorrhea). Soon to be licensed for sale are tobramycin (virtually identical with gentamicin) and amikacin (possessing attributes of both kanamycin and gentamicin). The structural formulas of these drugs are given in Figure 3-1.

With the exception of spectinomycin, these aminocyclitols are also aminoglycosides, i.e., glycosidically linked aminosugars are components of the molecules: either streptidine (as in streptomycin) or deoxystreptamine (as in kanamycin, gentamicin, tobramycin, and amikacin). However, macrolide and polyene antimicrobics are also aminoglycosides, e.g., desosamine in erythromycin (Fig. 3-6) and mycosamine in amphotericin B (Fig. 3-17). Thus, "aminoglycoside" is far too broad a term; "aminocyclitol" is suitably restrictive.

The aminocyclitols are fermentation products of *Streptomyces* spp. (streptomycin, kanamycin, spectinomycin) and *Micromonospora* spp. (gentamicin, tobramycin); amikacin is a semi-synthetic aminocyclitol derived from kanamycin.

Generally prepared as sulfates, the aminocyclitols are readily soluble in water. The stability of solutions decreases as the pH and/or the temperature is increased. Oxidizing and reducing agents also inactivate aminocyclitols. There is virtually no catabolism of aminocyclitols in man.

The primary mechanism of action involves intercalation of aminocyclitol molecules into messenger RNA (at sites that appear to be characteristic for each drug) of the 30 S ribosome; faulty transcription results. The proteins that are synthesized are nonfunctional and cell death follows. Mutations that block binding, or otherwise render it ineffective, lead to one-step, complete resistance.

A secondary mechanism relates to the abundant primary amino groups of kanamycin, gentamicin, tobramycin, and amikacin. The cationicity of these drugs is sufficient to yield a surface-active capability that contributes to antibacterial activity. Resistance to this detergent-like action occurs slowly if at all.

Table 3-1. Classification and Spectrum of Some Antimicrobics in Current Clinical Use

Chemical Class	Antimicrobic	Molecular Wt. (Free Base or Acid)	Activity Spectrum; Microbial Groups
Aminocyclitol	Streptomycin	581.6	
	Kanamycin	484.5	
	Gentamicin	447.6	*Narrow*
	Spectinomycin	332.4	Antibacterial
	Tobramycin	467.5	
	Amikacin	585.6	
Chloramphen- icol	Chloramphenicol	323.1	*Broad* Antichlamydial, antimyco- plasmal antirickettsial, and antibacterial
Ethambutol	Ethambutol	204.3	*Narrow* Antibacterial
Imidazole	Miconazole	479.2	*Broad* Antibacterial and antifungal
Lincomycin	Clindamycin	441.0	*Broad* Antibacterial and antiprotozoal
Macrolide	Erythromycin	733.9	*Broad* Antichlamydial, antimyco- plasmal, and antibacterial
	Rifampin	823.0	*Broad* Antiviral and antibacterial
Nitrofuran	Nitrofurantoin	238.2	*Narrow* Antibacterial
Organic Acids	Isonicotinic hydrazide	137.1	*Narrow* Antibacterial
	Mandelic	152.2	
	Nalidixic	232.2	

In addition to mutation to resistance through eliminating errors of transcription, bacteria may acquire plasmids encoding the synthesis of enzymes capable of inactivating aminocyclitols—either through adenylation, phosphorylation, or acetylation at specific key sites.

For systemic distribution, all the aminocyclitols must be injected. Intramuscular injection is well tolerated, and judicious intravenous injection is safe. Entry into the cerebrospinal fluid (CSF)

Table 3-1. Continued

Chemical Class	Antimicrobic	Molecular Wt. (Free Base or Acid)	Activity Spectrum; Microbial Groups
Peptide	Benzylpenicillin (G)	333.4	
	Phenoxymethyl penicillin (V)	350.4	
	Methicillin	380.4	
	Oxacillin	419.4	
	Cloxacillin	435.9	
	Dicloxacillin	471.3	
	Nafcillin	414.5	
	Ampicillin	349.4	*Narrow*
	Amoxacillin	419.4	Antibacterial
	Carbenicillin	368.4	
	Cephalothin	396.4	
	Cephaloridine	415.5	
	Cefazolin	454.5	
	Cephalexin	347.4	
	Polymyxin B	1,150	
	Polymyxin E	1,120	
Polyene	Amphotericin B	960.3	*Broad* Antiviral, antimycoplasmal, antifungal, and antiprotozoal
Pyrimidine	5-Fluorocytosine	129.1	*Broad* Antibacterial and antifungal
	Trimethoprim	290.3	*Broad* Antibacterial and antiprotozoal
Sulfonamide	Sulfadiazine	250.3	
	Sulfamerizine	264.3	*Broad*
	Sulfamethazine	278.4	Antichlamydial, antibacterial,
	Sulfisoxazole	267.3	and antiprotozoal
	Sulfamethoxazole	253.3	
Tetracycline	Oxytetracycline	460.2	*Broad*
	Tetracycline	444.2	Antichlamydial, antirickettsial
	Doxycycline	444.2	antimycoplasmal, and
	Minocycline	457.2	antibacterial

is negligible in the normal person. When there is a meningitis, streptomycin and possibly kanamycin, but not gentamicin (there are no data regarding the other aminocyclitols) attain therapeutic concentrations in the CSF.

As it is used in treating gonorrhea, spectinomycin does not appear to be toxic. The other aminocyclitols are potentially toxic for: (1) the eighth cranial nerves (vestibular toxicity with all; auditory toxicity uncommon with streptomycin but not uncommon with all others) and (2) the renal tubules (but rarely with streptomycin). Because these drugs are excreted primarily by the kidneys (glomerular filtration), renal dysfunction may lead to dangerous accumulation unless the dose is lowered to compensate for diminished excretory capacity.

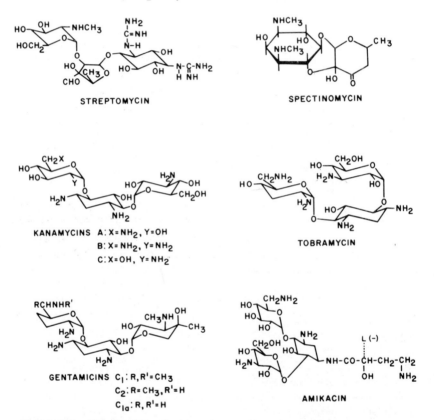

Figure 3-1. Structural formulas of aminocyclitol antimicrobics of current interest. Commercial kanamycin is primarily kanamycin A; gentamicin consists of approximately equal proportions of C_1, C_2, and C_{1a}.

CHLORAMPHENICOL

Chloramphenicol has two centers of optical activity (Fig. 3-2). Through synthesis of all possible enantiomorphs, the critical requirement for the structure exactly as elaborated by *Streptomyces venezuelae* was established. The drug in clinical use is produced by chemical synthesis.

The free base is poorly soluble in water but is well absorbed from the gut—after a given oral dose, the peak blood levels are about

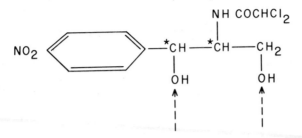

Figure 3-2. Chloramphenicol has two optically active carbon atoms (marked by asterisks). The drug can be inactivated by acetylation at the sites indicated by the arrows.

two-thirds as high as would be attained after injection of an identical dose. The succinate derivative is satisfactory for intramuscular and intravenous injection although the lag from injection to attainment of maximal concentration is prolonged by the need for hydrolytic cleavage of the chloramphenicol succinate complex. As ordinarily encountered, physical agents, such as heat, light, pH, and oxygen, have little deleterious effect.

In susceptible bacteria, chloramphenicol blocks protein synthesis through inhibition of extension of peptide chains undergoing synthesis in 50 S ribosomes. Although direct proof is lacking, it is assumed that inhibition of growth of nonbacterial microorganisms that are susceptible to chloramphenicol comes about in the same way.

Resistance to chloramphenicol may occur through inactivation of the drug by acetylation. The genetic information enabling synthesis of acetylating enzymes is acquired by gram-negative bacilli through transfer of the appropriate plasmid. There is also an innate resistance that does not involve inactivation of chloramphenicol and may reflect impermeability to the antimicrobic; such intrinsic resistance is encountered more often in gram-positive than in gram-negative bacteria.

Only about one-tenth of a dose of chloramphenicol is excreted as active drug in the urine; hepatic catabolism (hydrolysis; conjugation with glucuronic acid) inactivates the remainder, and the metabolites are excreted in the urine. The active drug does not accumulate in renal failure; the hepatic capacity for catabolism apparently accommodates to an increased supply. Chloramphenicol readily accumulates to toxic concentrations in premature and newborn infants because of their underdeveloped ability to conjugate chloramphenicol and their low renal excretory capacity. Chloramphenicol distributes readily throughout the body, including the central nervous system.

Interference with protein synthesis may also occur in man, with the severity of manifestations directly proportional to the dose. Such direct, dose-related toxicity typically causes anemia, leukopenia, and thrombocytopenia. Reversion to normal is complete when the drug is withdrawn. Quite in contrast is the rare bone marrow aplasia, in which there is apparently no relation to dose and the probability of reversal is low.

ETHAMBUTOL

Ethambutol is a product of chemical synthesis that has moderate activity against *Mycobacterium tuberculosis* (Fig. 3-3). It is a secondary drug that is given along with a primary agent, e.g.,

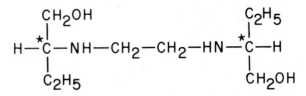

Figure 3-3. Ethambutol has two optically active carbon atoms (marked by asterisks). Only the dextro-isomer has anti-tuberculous activity.

isonicotinic acid hydrazide (INH), to forestall the emergence of INH-resistant tubercle bacilli. The drug is stable to heat. It is available only for oral administration. As the dihydrochloride, about 15% of the dose is catabolized to inactive end products in normal man.

The mechanism (or mechanisms) of action has not been defined. Because inhibition is not evident until two or three cell divisions have occurred, the drug may block generation of an essential metabolite. Resistance develops slowly under *in vivo* experimental conditions, and through mechanisms that are unknown.

Ethambutol is efficiently absorbed after peroral administration. Although entry into erythrocytes has been documented, there does not seem to be accumulation in other tissues. Urinary excretion is primary; although there is excretion in the feces, it is not clear whether biliary clearance is involved or not.

A dose-related optic neuritis is the major toxic effect of ethambutol. The process is reversible if the drug is withdrawn soon after the onset of symptoms.

MICONAZOLE

An imidazole derivative (Fig. 3-4), miconazole is an antifungal agent produced by chemical synthesis. It is insoluble in water but

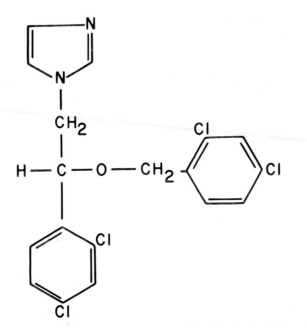

Figure 3-4. Miconazole is one of a series of imidazole derivatives that have antimycotic activity.

soluble in lipids and lipid solvents. Absorption from the gut is poor. As an aqueous suspension stabilized with polyethoxylated castor oil, the drug may be injected intravenously for systemic therapy.

Antifugal activity is unaffected by exposure to 37°C for one week in aqueous systems. Likewise, light, nonphysiologic pHs, and oxygen are not deleterious.

Fungistasis is the usual effect at concentrations that are clinically relevant. The way in which the drug acts is unknown.

Natively resistant strains among pathogenic fungi are rare. Development of resistance either in the laboratory or during therapy has not been reported.

In man, a non-adaptive hepatic catabolism rapidly degrades the drug following intravenous injection. A metabolite that appears in the urine, 2,5-dichloromandelic acid, accounts for about 25% of the dose. The drug does not accumulate when there is renal failure. Low, generally subtherapeutic, concentrations of antifungally active drug are attained in the urine and CSF.

Aside from such dose-related effects as giddiness, nausea, and vomiting, the drug may cause thrombophlebitis and is quite irritating to tissues if inadvertently injected outside a vein. Allergic reactions have been encountered.

CLINDAMYCIN

Clindamycin is a semi-synthetic derivative of lincomycin (Fig. 3-5). As the free base, it is insoluble in water; the hydrochloride and other salts are water soluble. The drug is well absorbed after

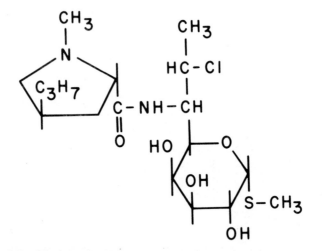

Figure 3-5. Clindamycin, 7-chloro-lincomycin, is better absorbed from the gut than the parent compound, lincomycin.

oral administration and may also be injected intramuscularly or intravenously. Clindamycin may be inactivated by heating. Catabolism does not appear to be extensive in man.

In susceptible bacteria, there appears to be a decrease in the synthesis of protein. The mechanism (or mechanisms) of anti-protozoal action, e.g., against *Plasmodium* spp., is even less well known. One-step mutation to high-level resistance has been observed with *Staphylococcus aureus*, but has not been reported with the nonsporulating anaerobes.

Systemic distribution does not extend to the central nervous system in the absence of meningitis. Excretion in the bile exceeds that in the urine, and no adjustment in dosage is required when there is renal failure.

Although loose stools, even diarrhea, are not uncommon, the serious adverse reaction is enterocolitis—a complication that may occur after parenteral therapy. Allergy is a rare occurrence.

ERYTHROMYCIN

The first of the macrolide antimicrobics to come to wide clinical use, erythromycin base (Fig. 3-6) is poorly soluble in water. However, several derivations are available: (1) oral administration of a

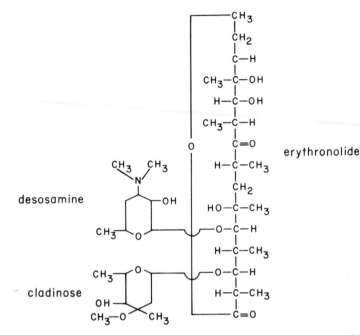

Figure 3-6. Erythromycin, a fermentation product of *Str. erythreus*, contains the glycosidically linked aminohexose, desosamine. Therefore, it is an aminoglycosidic macrolide antimicrobic.

simple salt, such as the stearate, results in poor absorption— comparable to the free base, (2) esterification to yield the propion- ate or the ethylsuccinate makes for more efficient absorption from the gut, and (3) either the lactobionate or the glucoheptonate salts are suitable for intravenous, but not intramuscular, injection. The drug may be inactivated by heating and is unstable at acid pH. Catabolism in man is not extensive.

Protein synthesis is blocked in the 30 S ribosome of susceptible bacteria. Although chlamydias and mycoplasmas have not been studied in comparable detail, it is assumed that erythromycin acts in the same way against these microorganisms.

Resistance has not been shown to involve destruction of the drug. With S. *aureus*, one-step mutation to a high level of resistance has been observed both during treatment and in the laboratory.

Systemic distribution excludes the central nervous system unless there is a meningitis. In the normal patient, the primary route of excretion is in the bile. When renal function is compromised, the dose need not be altered as the biliary excretory capacity readily accommodates to the small increase in load (only about 5% appears in the urine in normal patients).

Loose stools and increased frequency of defecation are common side-effects of treatment with erythromycin. The esterified forms of the drug have been associated with hepatic dysfunction that may vary in severity from that causing transient, mild anorexia to that provoking icterus; recovery is complete after withdrawal of the drug.

RIFAMPIN

One of several semi-synthetic derivatives of rifamycin B, rifampin (Fig. 3-7) is available only in a form suitable for oral administration. It is not excessively labile to heat but it is readily oxidized; it

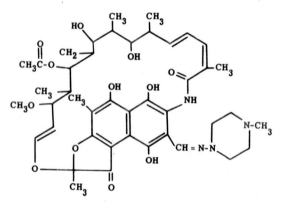

Figure 3-7. Rifampin is approved for use only in tuberculosis therapy and for the chemoprophylaxis of meningococcal meningitis.

is more stable at acid than alkaline pH. Catabolism has not been shown to occur in man.

DNA-dependent RNA polymerase is blocked by rifampin. In DNA viruses, nucleic acid synthesis is inhibited.

Massive resistance may develop as a one-step acquisition, particularly with *S. aureus* and *Mycobacterium tuberculosis*. Consequently, rifampin must always be used with another, effective, drug. The nature of the resistance has not been defined.

There is meager entry of rifampin into the central nervous system, even when there is meningitis. Biliary excretion and urinary excretion are both active in the normal patient. Although there is reabsorption after biliary excretion, there is no need to reduce the dose of rifampin when there is renal failure.

Hepatic dysfunction has been attributed to rifampin.

NITROFURANTOIN

Nitrofurantoin (Fig. 3-8) is one of several nitrofurans—all produced by chemical synthesis—that have antibacterial activity.

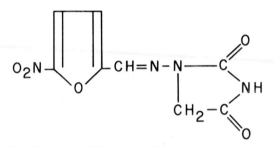

Figure 3-8. Nitrofurantoin attains clinically useful concentrations only in the urine.

Rarely injected (a sodium derivative is suitable for intravenous injection), the drug is usually given by mouth. It is a stable compound under physiologic conditions and does not appear to be susceptible to catabolism. It is light sensitive. The mechanism of action of nitrofurantoin on susceptible bacteria has not been defined. Resistance does occur and appears to be intrinsic, native, and undefined as to mechanism; it is not dependent on inactivation of the drug.

Nitrofurantoin is almost completely absorbed from the gut and is cleared by the kidneys so efficiently that there is no systemic distribution. After intravenous injection, the drug is only transiently detectable in the blood. Because of virtually total dependence on renal clearance for elimination, nitrofurantoin is not recommended for use when there is renal failure.

Except for the rare occurrence of allergy, toxicity from nitrofurantoin given in normal dosage is restricted to patients with impaired renal excretory ability.

Polyneuropathy and an interstitial pneumonitis are recognized toxic adverse reactions.

ISONICOTINIC ACID

Synthesized and prepared as the hydrazide, hence referred to as INH, the drug is a ligand capable of chelating divalent cations (Fig. 3-9). It may interfere with metabolic events requiring pyridoxal as a cofactor e.g., transaminases.

Native resistance in *M. tuberculosis* was present at the time INH was introduced into therapy. With worldwide use, the frequency of native resistance has increased measurably but slightly. Resistance has not been shown to involve alteration or destruction of the drug.

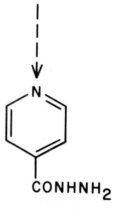

Figure 3-9. Isonicotinic acid hydrazide (INH) is produced by chemical synthesis. Acetylation (site indicated by arrow) inactivates the drug.

Because mutation to resistance in *M. tuberculosis* occurs once in approximately 10^7 replications, INH should never be used as the sole agent in therapy. However, it may be used alone in chemoprophylaxis when the body burden of tubercle bacilli is low and the cell mediated defenses are primed.

Absorption from the gut is quantitative, and the drug is distributed wherever there is water, i.e., there is no barrier to entry into the central nervous system. Acetylation, referred to above, occurs in the liver. Excretion is primarily through the kidney; however, the dose need not be decreased when there is renal failure because hepatobiliary excretion increases compensatorily.

Neurotoxicity from INH can be avoided by concomitant administration of pyridoxine. Hepatotoxicity varies in severity from the nonclinical—detected only by elevation in the concentrations of transaminases of hepatic origin—to jaundice and liver failure.

MANDELIC ACID

An aromatic organic acid (Fig. 3-10) that is not catabolizable, mandelic acid is also stable to physical agents such as heat, light,

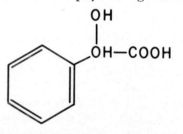

Figure 3-10. Mandelic acid is used as the racemate and is often prescribed as a "salt" compounded with hexamethylenamine tetraamine.

and oxygen. Limited in use to the treatment of urinary tract infections, mandelic acid is compounded with hexamethylenamine tetraamine for oral administration.

Susceptible bacteria are killed by mandelic acid through undefined mechanisms. Because the drug gains entry into bacterial cells only when it is un-ionized, it is effective only at an acid pH. It is useful only for the treatment of lower urinary tract infections, provided the pH of the urine can be maintained at or below 5.5.

Native resistance occurs and is usual among gram-positive bacteria. Acquisition of resistance during therapy has not been reported.

Absorption of orally administered mandelic acid is excellent. The drug is rapidly cleared by the kidneys—apparently the only excretory route—and there is virtually no systemic distribution. The drug is not ordinarily used when renal function is compromised. A metabolic acidosis may result if mandelic acid accumulates.

NALIDIXIC ACID

A product of chemical synthesis, nalidixic acid (Fig. 3-11) is stable to heat, light, and oxygen. It is rapidly metabolized in the human to yield products without antimicrobial activity.

The mechanism of action of nalidixic acid on susceptible bacteria is not known.

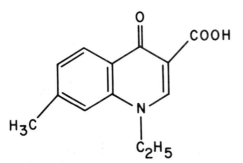

Figure 3-11. Nalidixic acid is a naphthyridine derivative. Antibacterial activity does not appear to be a function of pH.

Native resistance is infrequent among gram-negative bacteria. However, the emergence of high-level resistance as a single-step acquisition is so frequent as to limit the therapeutic utility of this drug. The mechanism of resistance is not known; it does not appear to involve destruction of alteration of nalidixic acid.

Following oral administration, nalidixic acid is absorbed, metabolized nearly completely, and then excreted by the kidneys—about 85% of the drug that appears in the urine has no antibacterial activity. Renal excretory capacity is high; all of the drug, active or not, that is delivered in the afferent blood is removed.

Nausea, vomiting, and allergic skin rashes have been reported as adverse reactions to nalidixic acid.

PENICILLINS

The characteristic nucleus of the penicillins results from the bicyclization of the dipeptide *l*-cysteinyl-*l*-valine (Fig. 3-12). In the

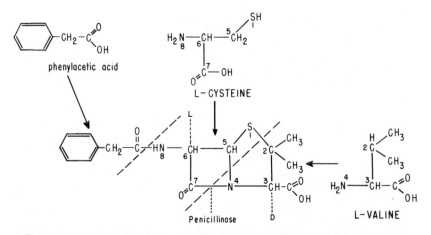

Figure 3-12. Benzylpenicillin, penicillin G, results when the bicyclic dipeptide, formed by condensation of *l*-valine with *l*-cysteine, is acylated with phenylacetic acid. The optical configuration at C-3 is inverted in the process of condensation (*dashed arrow*). Hydrolysis by β-lactamases, e.g. staphylococcal penicillinase, inactivates the drug (*dotted arrow*). (From P. D. Hoeprich. 1968. Calif. Med. *109*:301-308.)

process, there is inversion of the optical activity of C-3 to the *d* configuration. This inversion to an "unnatural" optical configuration was proved to be utterly essential to antibacterial activity when all possible enantiomorphs of penicillin V were synthesized. Acylation of the nucleus at the 6-amino position is the final step in the synthesis of the various penicillins either by *Penicillium* spp. or by the chemist. The addition of substituents at the 6-amino position appears to be the only manipulation that can be carried out with preservation of antibacterial activity. Thus, the various penicillins, natural and semi-synthetic, are characterized by the "side-chains" attached to the 6-amino group. The substituents of the penicillins referred to in this discussion are listed in Figure 3-13.

GENERIC NAME	SUBSTITUENT AT 6-AMINO	
	CHEMICAL NAME	STRUCTURE
Penicillin G	benzyl–	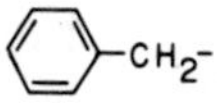
Penicillin V	phenoxymethyl–	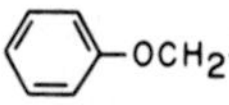
Methicillin	dimethoxyphenyl–	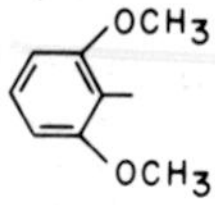
Oxacillin	5–methyl–3–phenyl–4–isoxazolyl–	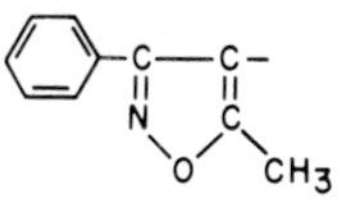
Cloxacillin	5–methyl–3–o–chlorophenyl–4–isoxazolyl–	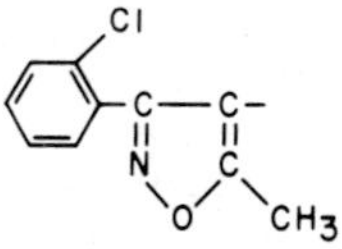
Dicloxacillin	5–methyl–3–o–dichlorophenyl–4–isoxazolyl–	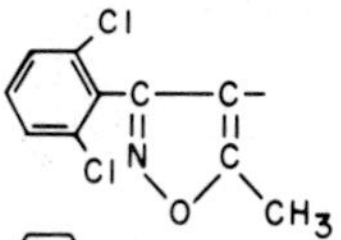
Nafcillin	6–(2–ethoxy–1)–napthamido–	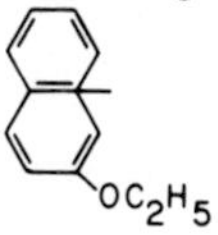
Ampicillin	alpha–aminobenzyl–	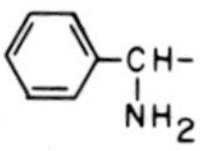
Amoxacillin	alpha–amino–para–hydroxybenzyl–	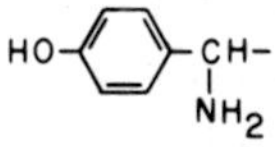
Carbenicillin	alpha–carboxybenzyl–	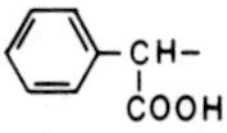

Figure 3-13. "Side-chains" characteristic of several penicillins.

The three goals of semi-synthesis were to provide penicillins that are: (1) resistant to acid, (2) resistant to β-lactamases, and (3) altered in antibacterial spectrum.

1. Resistance to Acid. Among natural penicillins, phenoxymethylpenicillin (penicillin V) was remarkable in surviving exposure to acid much better than benzylpenicillin (penicillin G). Semi-synthetic penicillins vary widely in resistance to degradation by acid; the relative resistance of pencillins to acid is shown in Table 3-2. These data provide a ready explanation for the utility of

Table 3-2. Comparative Resistance of Penicillins to Acid and Penicillinase

Penicillin	Resistance* to	
	Acid	Penicillinase
Penicillin G	2.5	5
Penicillin V	70	5
Methicillin	0.5	100
Oxacillin	70	80
Cloxacillin	70	80
Dicloxacillin	70	80
Nafcillin	70	80
Ampicillin	100	5
Amoxacillin	100	5
Carbenicillin	5	5

* Expressed as relative values: 100 = maximal resistance and 0 = total susceptibility.

penicillin V, cloxacillin, dicloxacillin, ampicillin, and amoxacillin. It is equally clear why penicillin G, methicillin, and carbenicillin are poorly absorbed after oral administration. Although oxacillin and nafcillin are relatively resistant to acid, for reasons that are unclear there is marked variation in efficiency of absorption. Ampicillin is quite resistant to acid, but attains relatively low concentrations in the blood after oral administration as compared with injection—most likely because efficient hepatobiliary excretion sequesters ampicillin in an enterohepatic cycle.

2. *Resistance to β-Lactamases.* As is indicated in Table 3-2, methicillin, the isoxazolyl penicillins (oxacillin, cloxacillin, dicloxacillin) and nafcillin are resistant to hydrolysis by those β-lactamases that are active against penicillin G. It is important to note that penicillin V, ampicillin, amoxacillin, and carbenicillin are quite susceptible to such β-lactamases.

3. *Altered Antibacterial Spectrum.* Ampicillin has significantly greater activity than penicillin G against *Hemophilus influenzae*, the enterococcal group of streptococci, *Salmonella typhi*, and most strains of *Escherichia coli* and *Proteus mirabilis*. Amoxacillin appears to be similarly altered in antibacterial effectiveness.

Carbenicillin is active not only against *Pseudomonas aeruginosa* but also against the indole-positive *Proteus* spp. and the *Providencia* spp.

All the penicillins are fragile compounds that undergo spontaneous decomposition even as apparently dry powders. Although they are not catabolized in man, spontaneous decomposition continues at body temperature and pH.

All the penicillins have a common mechanism of action: competitive inhibition of polymerization of sub-units of the bacterial cell wall. Because nonbacterial life forms either do not have cell walls or, as with fungi, have cell walls that differ in composition from bacteria, the penicillins are virtually restricted in activity to the bacteria. Antibacterial activity is most pronounced against the majority of gram-positive genera, the gram-negative cocci, and a few gram-negative bacilli.

Not all bacteria are susceptible to the penicillins. Resistance may depend on elaboration of β-lactamases that destroy the activity of penicillins (elaborated by both gram-positive and gram-negative bacteria). There is, in addition, resistance that does not involve destruction or alteration of the penicillin molecule. Such tolerance, or indifference, has not been explained.

Penicillins enter all body fluids readily, except those of the central nervous system, the eyes, the upper respiratory tract, and the prostate. Because the penicillins are so well tolerated, it is possible to achieve such high concentrations in the blood that barrier mechanisms may fail to exclude penicillins from these fluids. Also, inflammation (e.g., meningitis) reduces the effectiveness of barriers to entry of penicillins.

Penicillins are excreted primarily through the kidneys, by both glomerular filtration and tubular secretion. Tubular secretory capability can be competitively overcome by the concurrent administration of probenecid. Penicillin G, penicillin V, and methicillin are excreted almost exclusively by the kidneys. When there is renal failure, and/or if the dose is excessive, these penicillins may attain toxic concentrations. The isoxazolyl penicillins, as well as nafcillin, ampicillin, amoxacillin, and carbenicillin, are excreted sufficiently well by the liver to provide a safety valve against accumulation of these penicillins when renal function is reduced.

When very high concentrations are attained, i.e., in excess of 200 μg/ml serum, sufficient penicillin to cause intoxication may enter the central nervous system. Muscular twitching, confusion, even seizures, may result. Withdrawal of the drug leads to disappearance of the toxicity.

The major adverse reaction is hypersensitivity. Overall, penicillins may be the commonest causes of drug allergies, even as they are among the most commonly prescribed drugs. When anti-penicillin antibodies of the IgE class circulate in the plasma, absorption of a penicillin (any penicillin) will provoke an immediate, anaphylactoid reaction that may be fatal. Late or delayed reactions in the form of skin rashes are much more common.

An interstitial nephritis has been associated with the use of methicillin. Toxic injury to the bone marrow, manifested as agranulocytosis or aplasia, is another adverse reaction that may be caused by methicillin.

CEPHALOSPORINS

The characteristic nucleus of the cephalosporins results from the bicyclization of the dipeptide formed from *l*-cysteine with α,β-dehydro,γ-hydroxyvaline (Fig. 3-14). Two sites are available for

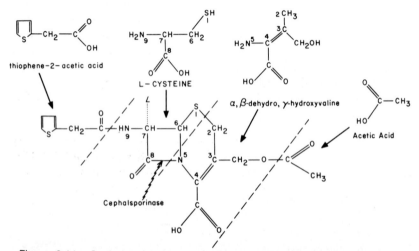

Figure 3-14. Cephalothin is a semi-synthetic antimicrobic that results from (1) acylation of the amino group at C-7 with thiophene-2-acetic acid and (2) esterification of the methanolic -OH at C-3 with acetic acid. The cephalosporin nucleus is elaborated by *Cephalosporium acremonium* through condensation of *l*-cysteine with α,β-dehydro,γ-hydroxyproline. β-lactamases, as formed by many gram-negative bacilli, attack the β-lactam ring at the site indicated by the arrow.

modification: the amino group at C-7 (analogous to the amino group of C-6 of the penicillins) and a methanolic -OH at C-3. All the cephalosporins useful to therapy are semi-synthetic compounds prepared by acylation and esterification of the nucleus which is derived from cephalosporin C, a fermentation product of *Cephalosporium acremonium*. The formulas of the other cephalosporins referred to in this chapter are listed in Figure 3-15. In addition to antibacterial activity, desirable pharmacologic properties, such as good absorption after oral administration and stability *in vitro*, have been attained.

All the cephalosporins are relatively fragile compounds that decompose spontaneously on storage and are heat labile. Although somewhat more tolerant of deviations from physiologic pH than

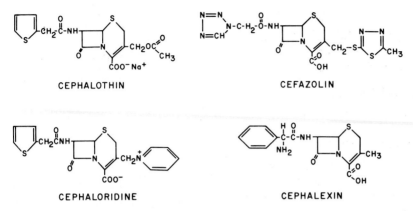

CEPHALOTHIN

CEFAZOLIN

CEPHALORIDINE

CEPHALEXIN

Figure 3-15. Although the number of cephalosporins on the market has steadily increased, several of the newer congeners offer no advantages. Thus, cephapirin is equivalent to cephalothin, and cephradine is equivalent to cephalexin. Although cefazolin has much the same pharmacokinetics as cephaloridine, nephrotoxicity has not been associated with cefazolin. However, unlike cephaloridine, cefazolin does not enter the cerebrospinal fluid.

some of the penicillins, extremes speed decomposition. Those cephalosporins esterified with acetic acid at the methanolic -OH of C-3 are susceptible to inactivation by deacetylation in the liver (and possibly kidneys): cephalothin, cephapirin, cephaloglycin.

The mechanism of antibacterial action of the cephalosporins is identical with that of the penicillins: inhibition of cell-wall synthesis.

Resistance is also analogous in that certain β-lactamases elaborated by gram-negative bacteria are capable of hydrolyzing the β-lactam ring of the cephalosporins. However, the β-lactamases of *Staphylococcus aureus* are inactive against most cephalosporins. There is also an intrinsic resistance of undefined nature that does not involve destruction or alteration of the cephalosporins.

The distribution of the cephalosporins in the body is, once again, generally analogous to that of the penicillins. However, except for cephaloridine, none of the cephalosporins penetrate into the cerebrospinal fluid in therapeutically adequate quantities, regardless of inflammation of the meninges or of dosage.

The cephalosporins are excreted primarily through the kidneys. Both glomerular filtration and tubular secretion (except for cephaloridine) occur; tubular secretion may be blocked by the simultaneous administration of probenecid. Cephaloridine appears to be reabsorbed in the proximal convoluted tubules of the kidney.

The major adverse reactions to the cephalosporins are those of hypersensitivity. There does not appear to be true cross-hypersensitivity between penicillins and cephalosporins. However, as with other drug allergies, persons allergic to the penicillins are more likely to develop allergy to the cephalosporins than are non-allergic persons.

Three cephalosporins provoke inordinate pain on intramuscular injection: cephalothin, cephapirin, and cephacetrile. These agents also tend to cause thrombophlebitis on intravenous injection.

Two cephalosporins have potential for nephrotoxicity that can be avoided by judicious dosage: cephaloridine and cephacetrile.

POLYMYXINS

Products of *Bacillus polymyxa*, non-Actinomycete bacteria, the polymyxins are cyclic decapeptides subtending multiple primary amines from diaminobutyric acid moieties (Fig. 3-16). Polymyxin B

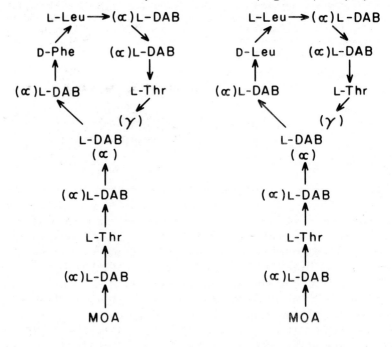

The (α) and (γ) designations indicate that the respective NH_2 groups are involved in the peptide linkages.
DAB = α,γ-diaminobutyric acid residue
MOA = (+)-6-methyloctanoic acid residue.

Figure 3-16.   Of the five recognized polymyxins (A-E), only polymyxins B and E have come to therapeutic application, E under the name colistin. At present, these agents have been replaced by gentamicin and carbenicillin.

and polymyxin E (colistin) are two polymyxins of therapeutic importance; each has six primary amino groupings. Both compounds are relatively stable to physiologic temperature and pH; they are not susceptible to catabolism in man. They are soluble in water.

For systemic therapy, the polymyxins must be injected— polymyxin B as the sulfate, polymyxin E as the anionic methanesulfonate derivative. Polymyxin E methanesulfonate is intrinsically inactive to the extent that its amino groups have been converted by sulfomethylation to anionic moieties. Hydrolysis occurs spontaneously in aqueous systems at physiologic pH to release the active drug. Both drugs may be given by mouth, as the sulfates, to suppress aerobic gram-negative bacillary flora.

The polymyxins are cationic surface active agents that disorganize cell membranes through combination with phospholipids. The particular activity of the polymyxins against *Pseudomonas aeruginosa* may reflect the relative richness of pseudomonal cell membranes in phospholipids.

Native resistance to the polymyxins occurs, e.g., among grampositive bacteria. However, the mechanism (or mechanisms) is not defined.

Since they are relatively large and highly charged molecules, the polymyxins fail to enter such special fluid compartments as the central nervous system, eye, upper respiratory tract, and prostate. The polymyxins are excreted in the urine by glomerular filtration.

POLYENES

The polyenes are among the most commonly elaborated antimicrobics of the soil-dwelling *Streptomyces* spp. When particular strains of *Streptomyces nodosus* are grown under the proper conditions, amphotericin B accumulates as a sludge on the mycelia. As other polyenes, amphotericin B is a large ring structure consisting of a rigid (unsaturated heptaene), hydrophobic portion and a flexible, hydrophilic (alcohol -OHs) portion (Fig. 3-17). There are two ionizable moieties: (1) a carboxyl at C-16, near the hydrophobichydrophilic junction of the ring and (2) a primary amine that is a substituent of mycosamine, a six-carbon aminosugar attached by a glycosidic bond to C-19 of the ring. As a consequence, amphotericin B is amphoteric—it is insoluble in water at physiologic pH. A suspension, stabilized with sodium deoxycholate, is used for therapy. The suspension is light sensitive and deteriorates rapidly in culture media, less rapidly in serum, less rapidly still in 0.9% NaCl or 5% glucose solutions. It is stable for a week at 37°C in distilled water. Amphotericin B is not catabolizable in man. Within

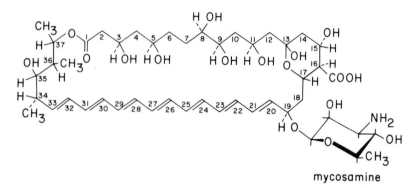

mycosamine

Figure 3-17. Amphotericin B is a heptaene that contains the glycosidically linked aminohexose, mycosamine. Therefore, it is an aminoglycosidic polyene antimicrobic.

minutes of exposure, amphotericin B interacts with sterols of susceptible eukaryotic cell membranes (exception: certain mycoplasmas), disorganizing the membrane so that K^+ is lost. As injury progresses, Mg^{++} escapes from the cell, followed in turn by amino acids; protein synthesis diminishes and the cell dies. There is some evidence that (1) amphotericin B has particular affinity for ergosterol and (2) phospholipids may also interact with amphotericin B.

Resistance to amphotericin B does occur among fungi. Strains of *Saccharomyces cerevisiae* selected in the laboratory for resistance have decreased ergostenane sterols and increased cholestenane sterols.

For systemic therapy, amphotericin B must be injected intravenously. There is limited passage out of the blood—no entry into the central nervous system. The primary route of excretion is hepatobiliary, with antifungally active drug in the bile. Glomerular filtration accounts for relatively little excretion.

Minor, reversible, adverse reactions include thrombophlebitis, nausea and vomiting, abdominal pain, chills, fever, and anorexia. Potentially lethal effects include: (1) nephrotoxicity—tubular injury, which probably results as the drug is concentrated as water is reabsorbed from the glomerular filtrate, (2) hypokalemia—most likely secondary to injury to the erythrocyte cell membrane, and (3) bone marrow depression. Azotemia, reduced renal functional capacity, and anemia are commonly seen. When subarachnoid injection of amphotericin B is required, arachnoiditis may be engendered in the region of the injection; diminished acuity of hearing may also result.

5-FLUOROCYTOSINE

Synthesized as a potential anti-cancer agent, 5-fluorocytosine (5-FC) is exactly what the name indicates—the pyrimidine cytosine with a fluorine atom at the 5-position of the ring (Fig. 3-18). The drug is quite stable to heat, light, acids, and alkalis.

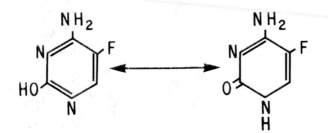

Figure 3-18. 5-Fluorocytosine is tautomeric in aqueous systems at physiologic pH.

Only microorganisms that depend on conversion of cytosine to uracil are susceptible to 5-FC. Of itself, 5-FC is innocuous to man; if it is oxidatively deaminated to yield 5-fluorouracil, it becomes potentially toxic—through incorporation into nucleic acids to cause miscoding that may result in serious injury to the cell.

Primary toxicity does not occur in man because humans do not have the enzymatic capability to convert 5-FC to 5-fluorouracil. If, however, 5-FC becomes available to the enteric microflora, bacterial synthesis of 5-fluorouracil may lead to toxicity (e.g., bone marrow depression) if sufficient 5-fluorouracil is absorbed.

Microbial resistance depends on utilization of noncytosine sources of uracil. Mutation to such resistance during therapy has been documented. Native resistance is widespread among fungi and may relate to the utilization of alternate pathways to uracil.

Commercially available as tablets for peroral administration, 5-FC is readily and efficiently absorbed from the gut. Distribution is general—into all body water. The drug is excreted, unchanged, by the kidneys. Renal failure leads to accumulation of the drug unless the dose is suitably reduced.

TRIMETHOPRIM

Conceived, designed, and synthesized in the research laboratories of the Burroughs Wellcome Company, trimethoprim is one of a series of 2,4-diaminopyrimidines (Fig. 3-19). It is distinguished from its congeners by particular activity against bacteria and moderate antiprotozoal activity. For therapy, it is available

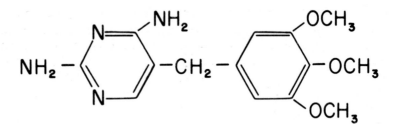

Figure 3-19. Trimethoprim is one compound of a family of 2,4-diaminopyrimidines. It has particular affinity for the dihydrofolate reductase of susceptible bacteria and thus competitively inhibits this essential enzyme.

mixed with sulfamethoxazole in a fixed ratio (1:20), pressed into a tablet for peroral administration. The compound is quite stable to the usual physical agents. It is soluble in water and is not susceptible to catabolism in man.

All the 2,4-diaminopyrimidines inhibit competitively dihydrofolate reductase. Trimethoprim exhibits an affinity for the bacterial enzyme that is at least 10^4 greater than its affinity for dihydrofolate reductase of human origin. Because dihydrofolate arises from condensation of glutamic acid with dihydropteroate and the dihydropteroate results from condensation of dihydropteridine with *p*-aminobenzoic acid (a sulfonamide-susceptible reaction), the possibility of synergy between trimethoprim and a sulfonamide was apparent. It has, in fact, been realized. These relationships are portrayed in Figure 3-20.

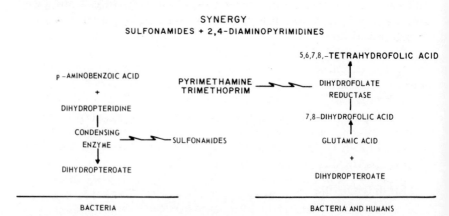

Figure 3-20. The basis for synergy between sulfonamides and 2,4-diaminopyrimidines rests on competitive inhibition of an essential sequence at two enzymatic loci. (From P. D. Hoeprich. 1968. Antimicrob. Agents Chemother. 7:697-704.)

Resistance to trimethoprim occurs and is of the intrinsic variety, i.e., neither destruction nor alteration of the antimicrobic is involved. Although it may not be a general mechanism in bacteria, resistance has been shown to result from elaboration of an isoenzyme—a dihydrofolate reductase that is, comparatively, little inhibited by trimethoprim. Another adaptation involves expansion of pathways that regenerate tetrahydrofolate.

Absorption from the gut is excellent. Trimethoprim attains higher concentrations in extravascular extracellular fluids than in the blood. Entry into the cerebrospinal fluid is meager. Renal excretion diminishes when there is renal dysfunction, and the drug may accumulate if the dose is not reduced.

When dosage is proper, there is no adverse effect from trimethoprim in man. Extraordinarily high concentrations, such as might result in a patient with renal failure if the dose were not reduced, might depress bone marrow function. Hypersensitivity occurs rarely if at all.

SULFONAMIDES

Steming from Domagk's epochal discovery of the antibacterial property of prontosil, sulfonamides have evolved through constant honing and refining of the molecule aimed at securing optimal pharmacologic properties. The five sulfonamides listed by chemical structure in Figure 3-21 may not include the ultimate sulfonamide, but they are drugs with properties insuring current use. All are available in tablet form for oral therapy; some, as sodium salts, are prepared as solutions for intramuscular or intravenous injection.

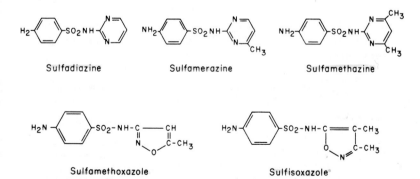

Figure 3-21. Some of the sulfonamides in current use are depicted above. Although pharmacokinetic properties vary greatly, all sulfonamides act on susceptible microorganisms in the same way.

Sulfadiazine, sulfamerazine, and sulfamethazine are, generically, sulfapyrimidines. In equal portions, they are prescribed as "triple sulfonamides," a mixture that has pharmacologic advantages of clinical importance. The solubility of each component in the urine is independent of the others, and so precipitation in the renal tubules is avoided. Sulfisoxazole and sulfamethoxazole are so soluble that they present no problem in this regard.

The sulfonamides are quite stable compounds. All are inactivated by the liver to a greater or lesser extent, depending on the drug. There is obliteration of the *p*-amino group by acetylation or glucuronidation. The conjugate may or may not be more soluble in water than the parent compound; generally, the conjugate is preferentially excreted by the kidneys.

All the sulfonamides act in the same way, namely, by competitive inhibition of synthesis of dihydropteroate (Fig. 3-20). Accordingly, all the sulfonamides are, potentially, capable of synergy with the 2,4-diaminopyrimidines. Thus, sulfadiazine in combination with pyrimethamine has been used successfully in the treatment of malaria and pneumocystosis. Sulfamethoxazole was paired with trimethoprim because the pharmacokinetics of the two drugs match so well: they have half-lives of 11 hours and 10.5 hours, respectively.

Native resistance to the sulfonamides appears to be explained by the discovery of an isoenzymic dihydropteroate synthetase in resistant bacteria. The isoenzyme has low affinity for sulfonamides and, comparatively, high affinity for the substrate *p*-aminobenzoic acid.

Sulfonamides distribute widely in body water entering the cerebrospinal fluid, eye, upper respiratory tract secretions, and, with derivatives of basic pK, prostate. Concentrations in the blood are usually higher than in extravascular fluids. Excretion is primarily in the urine. Of the drugs listed, sulfisoxazole is most rapidly excreted; indeed, it is difficult to obtain therapeutic concentrations of this sulfonamide outside the urinary tract. The sulfapyrimidines are less rapidly excreted, and six-hourly dosage results in maintenance of therapeutic concentrations in the blood (10-15 mg/100 ml). Sulfamethoxazole is even more slowly excreted—12-hourly dosage is generally adequate.

Nephrotoxicity of mechanical origin has been mentioned. The sulfonamides may also cause hypersensitivity. Hepatotoxicity, bone marrow depression—especially of the granulocyte series—hemolytic anemia, thyroiditis, and confusion are some of the other adverse reactions that have been observed. All are of reduced frequency of occurrence with the modern sulfonamides.

TETRACYCLINES

Oxytetracycline and tetracycline are fermentation products (*Streptomyces rimosus* and other species), whereas doxycycline and minocycline are semi-synthetic in origin. As is evident from inspection of the structural formulas (Fig. 3-22), oxytetracycline is the most polar of the group and minocycline is the least polar; lipophilicity varies accordingly.

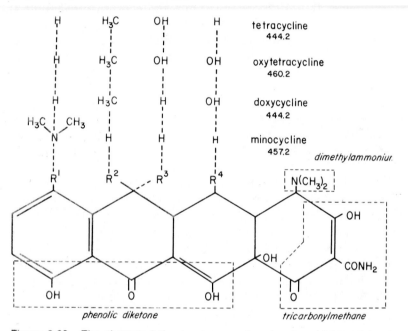

Figure 3-22. The characteristic structures and molecular weights of the four tetracyclines referred to in the text are indicated above. Dashed lines enclose the three ionizable microzones that comprise the inviolate regions of the tetracycline molecule. These microzones are not influenced in pKa to a biologically significant degree by the substituents, R_1-R_4, which distinguish the various congeners. (From P. D. Hoeprich. 1974. Antimicrob. Agents Chemother. 5:330-336.)

The tetracyclines are reasonably stable compounds although decompensation, even of the dry powder, will occur spontaneously over the period of a year. There is only minor catabolism of the tetracyclines in man. Preparations are available for oral and parenteral administration. Only about one-third of perorally administered oxytetracycline and tetracycline is absorbed, whereas absorption of both doxycycline and minocycline appears to be complete.

Inhibition of protein synthesis is agreed upon as the way in which tetracyclines inhibit bacterial growth. Precisely how this comes about is not known beyond the siting of action in the 50 S ribosome. Perhaps the avid chelating capability of the tetracyclines for divalent cations is important. It is assumed that nonbacterial microorganisms are affected in the same way as bacteria.

Resistance is well documented in bacteria, gram-positive and gram-negative alike. Destruction or modification of the drugs is not implicated. The mechanism (or mechanisms) is unknown.

With oxytetracycline, tetracycline, and, to a lesser extent, doxycycline, there is poor entry into the cerebrospinal fluid and the eye and upper respiratory tract secretions. Minocycline penetrates these liquids to a significantly greater extent. All the tetracyclines appear to enter sebum and keratinizing cells. Renal excretion is critical to elimination of oxytetracycline, tetracycline, and minocycline; these drugs accumulate if renal dysfunction is not compensated by reduction in dosage. Doxycycline, on the other hand, is not dependent on renal excretion and can be given in normal dosage to patients who are anephric. Although there is biliary excretion of tetracyclines, apparently reabsorption does occur.

Hypersensitivity to the tetracyclines is rare. Because they are strong ligands for divalent cations, the tetracyclines become incorporated in calcifying tissues. Although unsightly, the local effect can also be serious through inhibition of osteoid formation, leading to arrested bone growth and faulty dentition. Acute hepatic necrosis may be precipitated by tetracyclines, particularly in recently delivered women who are in shock. Outdated, that is, decomposed, tetracyclines may poison renal function, leading to glucosuria, aminoaciduria, and loss of electrolytes.

REFERENCES

1. Gottlieb, D., and P. D. Shaw, (Eds.). 1967. *Antibiotics I, Mechanisms of Action.* Springer-Verlag New York Inc., New York.
2. Hoeprich, P. D. (Ed.). 1972. *Infectious Diseases.* Harper & Row, Hagerstown, Maryland. pp. 177-205.
3. Todd, R. G. (Ed.). 1967. *Extra Pharmacopoeia Martindale.* 25th ed. The Pharmaceutical Press, London.
4. Umezawa, H. (Ed.). 1967. *Index of Antibiotics from Actinomycetes.* University Park Press, Baltimore, Md.

Section II
ANTIMICROBIC
DILUTION TESTS

Chapter 4

DILUTION TESTS:
GENERAL CONSIDERATIONS

Antimicrobic dilution tests are used to determine the minimal inhibitory concentration (MIC) or minimal lethal concentration (MLC), i.e., the lowest concentration of antimicrobic required to inhibit or "kill" a particular microorganism. Serial dilutions of the antimicrobial agent are incorporated into a nutrient broth or agar medium and then inoculated with a standardized suspension of the microorganism being tested. The primary advantage to such broth or agar dilution tests is that they permit a *quantitative* estimate of the activity of the antimicrobic.

In the clinical laboratory, *quantitative* susceptibility data are needed occasionally for proper management of chemotherapy, e.g., when drug dosage schedules must be monitored. Qualitative information provided by the disc diffusion test is usually adequate for guiding the therapy of most infections, but dilution tests are indicated when the disc test results are inapplicable, equivocal, or thought to be unreliable. For example, disc tests are inappropriate for testing slow-growing microorganisms, nutritionally fastidious strains, or microorganisms for which adequate standardization of disc methods has not yet been accomplished. With certain drugs the disc test is known to be unreliable or has not yet been adequately evaluated. In general, any strain that gives a zone falling into the equivocal, intermediate, category should be tested further by a dilution technique if an acceptable alternative drug is not available. In some situations, microorganisms that are categorized as being resistant by the disc diffusion technique might be treated preferentially and safely with massive doses of relatively nontoxic antimicrobics, such as the penicillins. Certain types of urinary tract infections might respond to therapy with ordinary doses of an antimicrobic that is concentrated within the urine, even though the microorganism is categorized as being intermediate or resistant by the disc test criteria. In these cases, a quantitative estimate of the degree of susceptibility of the microorganism might influence the choice of antimicrobic, the dose, or the route of administration. Broth dilution susceptibility tests are essential for testing combinations of two or more antimicrobic agents or for guiding therapy of an infection in which a bactericidal activity must be maintained, e.g., endocarditis.

Although the disc diffusion technique is usually adequate, the clinical laboratory should have the capacity to perform quantitative susceptibility tests with selected clinical isolates. Such procedures are cumbersome to perform and difficult to control adequately if they are performed only at infrequent, irregular intervals. For that reason, many microbiologists have found it desirable to adapt a dilution technique as the routine testing procedure. When a fairly large number of strains are being tested routinely, the agar dilution technique may be utilized by limiting the number of antimicrobic concentrations tested and by using an inoculum-replicating apparatus such as that described by Steers et al.[9] Broth dilution tests may be applied as a routine testing technique by use of microdilution procedures, with semi-automated equipment for preparing doubling dilutions of the drug. Whether the dilution test is to be used for special studies or as a routine procedure, the principles of the techniques remain the same (they are outlined in the following sections). Principles that apply equally to both agar and broth dilution techniques are as follows.

TEST MEDIUM

Selection of the most appropriate medium for antimicrobic dilution tests is at best a compromise. Although the ideal medium is not yet available, it should have the following characteristics:

1. The ideal medium must be capable of supporting growth of the majority of pathogens for which susceptibility tests are required, without additional enrichment.

2. The contents of the medium should be defined at least to the point of specific production details for crude components, such as "peptone" and agar.
3. Susceptibility test results should be reproducible on different batches of the medium prepared by different manufacturers.
4. The medium should be free of components known to be antagonistic to the common agents for which susceptibility tests are made.
5. The medium should not be subjected to marked shifts in pH, especially to the acid side, during growth of common pathogenic microorganisms.
6. The agar and broth versions of the medium should have the same formulation, except for the presence or absence of the solidifying agent.
7. The medium should be approximately isotonic for bacteria and the agar medium appropriate for addition of blood when required for growth of fastidious microorganisms.

Of the many media now available and commonly used for susceptibility testing, none meet all the requirements listed above. Several investigators have reported the development of chemically defined media that would approach more nearly the ideal for susceptibility testing. However, these media have not yet withstood the critical test of time. Because they are likely to be much more expensive, chemically defined media might be thought of only as standards for evaluating the performance of more complex undefined media, which, in turn, can be used for routine testing purposes.

For testing most rapid-growing bacterial pathogens, Mueller-Hinton medium is considered the best compromise. The broth and agar versions of this medium show rather good batch-to-batch reproducibility for susceptibility testing, are low in sulfonamide and tetracycline inhibitors, and give rather good growth of rapidly growing pathogens. For testing those strains that fail to grow adequately in this medium, the agar version can be supplemented by adding 5% (v/v) defibrinated sheep, horse, or human blood, provided that the blood has been found to be free of antimicrobial activity. Alternatively, the broth or agar medium may be supplemented with 5% (v/v) peptic digest of blood or 5% (v/v) laked horse or sheep blood (lysed by repeated freeze-thaw cycles and cleared of remnant cell stroma by centrifugation). Both the latter additives may be prepared in bulk and stored frozen until needed. For testing *Hemophilus* sp., the blood-containing agar medium may be "chocolatized" by heating to 80°C until the medium takes on a rich brown color, or better-defined sources of the X and V factors may be added.

Even with growth supplements, some microorganisms fail to grow adequately in a Mueller-Hinton medium. A medium such as a soy bean casein digest (tryptic or trypticase soy), agar or broth (without dextrose), or a similar medium may be used for testing nutritionally fastidious microorganisms, provided adequate controls are incorporated to demonstrate that the medium does not affect the activity of the antimicrobic being tested. This may be accomplished by testing one or more control strains along with the more fastidious microorganism in both the alternative medium and a Mueller-Hinton medium. The differences between the two MICs with the control strains provide information concerning the extent to which this departure from the standard medium might have affected the test strain.

The pH of the medium is one factor that markedly affects the activity of some antimicrobial agents (Table 4-1). In some media, the pH shifts rather dramatically as a result of microbial metabolism, especially when the test medium contains a fermentable carbohydrate. To demonstrate the extent to which pH shifts occur in some commonly used broth media, tubes were inoculated with the standard control strain of *Escherichia coli* and the pH was continually monitored for the first 24 hours of incubation (a semi-micro electrode and a pH meter attached to a continuous recording apparatus were used). The results are presented in Figure 4-1. In glucose-containing media, such as brain-heart infusion or trypticase soy broth, the pH fell rather dramatically and then returned toward neutrality as additional metabolic products accumulated and the intermediate organic acids were utilized. The shift in pH with Mueller-Hinton broth or trypticase soy broth without dextrose was much less dramatic and not as likely to influence the activity of antimicrobic agents. The synthetic amino-acid medium[4] resembled the fungal medium described in Figure 11-1, except that uracil was added (0.025 g/l) and the glucose reduced to 0.5 gm/l for testing bacteria. It contained two effective organic buffers (TRIS and MOPS) and thus the pH tended to remain quite stable during the

Table 4-1. Effect of pH on Antimicrobic Activity of Different Agents

Little Affected	Less Active in Acid Medium	Less Active in Alkaline Medium
Penicillin	Aminoglycosides	Tetracyclines
Chloramphenicol	Lincomycin	Methicillin
Polymyxins	Erythromycin	Cloxacillin
Vancomycin	group	Fucidin
	Cephaloridine	

SOURCE: L. P. Garrod, H. P. Lambert, F. O'Grady, and P. M. Waterworth. 1973. *Antibiotic and Chemotherapy*, 4th ed. Churchill Livingstone, Edinburgh. p. 493.

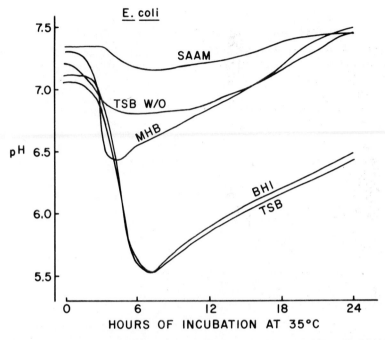

Figure 4-1. Shift in pH of five broth media during growth of *E. coli.* SAAM = Synthetic Amino Acid Medium (of Hoeprich et al.[4]); TSB W/O = trypticase soy broth without glucose; MHB = Mueller-Hinton broth; BHI = brain-heart infusion broth; TSB = trypticase soy broth. (From A. L. Barry, and L. J. Effinger. Unpublished data.)

entire period of incubation. For obvious reasons, a medium that demonstrates dramatic fluctuation in pH as a result of bacterial growth should not be selected for broth dilution testing and thus fermentable carbohydrates should be omitted except when essential for growth of the microorganism being tested. A similar pH change during the growth of *E. coli* on Mueller-Hinton agar is shown in Figure 4-2. The shift in pH is significantly affected by the atmospheric conditions under which the plate is incubated: an increased atmosphere of CO_2 produces an initial drop in the surface pH, but later an increase in pH results from the metabolic activity accompanying microbial growth.

At the time each batch of Mueller-Hinton medium is prepared, the pH should be checked with a pH meter. The medium should be between pH 7.2 and 7.4 at room temperature. If it is not, it may be adjusted with 0.1 N NaOH or 0.1 N HCl. Caution should be taken to avoid the addition of an excess of NaOH and back-titration with HCl since this would increase the concentration of Na and Cl, which, in turn, might affect certain antimicrobics. The pH of a medium is a function of its temperature (Fig. 4-3). The pH of Mueller-Hinton agar should be checked after gelling. The checking can be done by macerating a small amount of agar in a small volume of distilled water, or by allowing a small amount of agar to

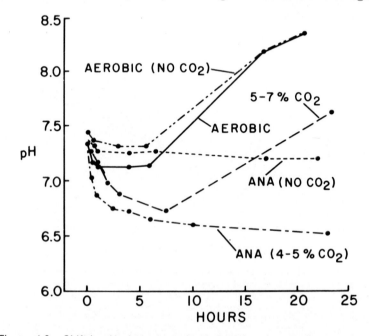

Figure 4-2. Shift in pH of Mueller-Hinton blood agar plates inoculated with *E. coli* and incubated under different atmospheric environments. (From J. E. Rosenblatt, and F. Schoenknecht. 1972. Antimicrob. Agents Chemother. *1:*435.)

solidify around a pH electrode in a beaker, or by using a properly calibrated surface electrode. If the pH is determined while the agar medium is still warm enough to be liquid, the temperature should be recorded and final pH adjusted accordingly.

The concentration of certain cations is critically important, especially when testing *Pseudomonas aeruginosa* against aminocyclitols. The final concentration of cations should be adjusted to yield from 20 to 35 mg of Mg^{++} per l and 50 to 100 mg of Ca^{++} per l, as determined by atomic absorption spectrophotometry.[6] Most Mueller-Hinton broth currently available commercially needs to be supplemented to obtain this cation concentration, but the agar version is usually satisfactory. Separate stock solution of $CaCl_2$ and of $MgCl_2$ may be prepared in concentrations that yield 10 mg of cation per ml. These stock solutions may be sterilized by passing them through a membrane filter and then adding appropriate volumes

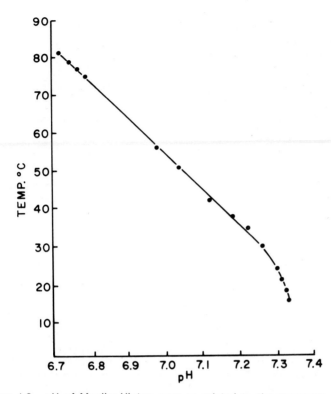

Figure 4-3. pH of Mueller-Hinton agar as related to the temperature of the medium. (From J. E. Rosenblatt and F. Schoenknecht. 1972. Antimicrob. Agents Chemother. *1:*435.)

aseptically to each batch of Mueller-Hinton broth after it has been autoclaved and allowed to cool to room temperature. The exact volume of salt solution required to bring the cation concentration to within acceptable ranges should be determined for each new lot of Mueller-Hinton agar or broth. The amount of variability that can be observed in different batches of media is displayed in Table 4-2, along with an estimate of the concentrations of magnesium and calcium normally found in serum.

PREPARATION OF ANTIMICROBIC STOCK SOLUTIONS

The preparation and maintenance of stock solutions of various antimicrobial agents is an extremely critical chore for the antimicrobic laboratory. Standard or reference preparations of antimicrobial agents can be obtained directly from the manufacturer, from commercial suppliers who provide testing powders specifically for susceptibility testing, or from the United States Pharmacopeia

(12601 Twinbrook Parkway, Rockville, Maryland 20852). Clinical preparations provided through the hospital pharmacy should not be used because they are less precisely standardized, often have other materials that might interfere with *in vitro* tests, and in some cases actually contain forms of the drug that are not active *in vitro*. For example, chloramphenicol sodium succinate cannot be used for *in vitro* testing since the ester develops full activity only after hydrolysis *in vivo*.

Antimicrobics for susceptibility testing are usually provided as dried powders and are labeled with an expiration date and a statement concerning the amount (μg or IU) of active substance per mg of powder. Unless otherwise specified by the supplier, the test powders should be stored at −20°C or lower and, if not sealed in glass ampules, the powders should be kept in a desiccator. A storage system must be developed to avoid continual opening and closing of the desiccator and repeated thawing and refreezing of the test powders.

Stock solutions are prepared in advance, usually in a concentration of 2,000 μg or IU/ml. This is accomplished by weighing a sample of the powder on an analytical balance and then dissolving it in an appropriate solvent. The actual weight of active substance in the sample is calculated by multiplying the weight of the sample (in mg) by the weight (μg or IU) of active substance per mg. The

Table 4-2. Total Concentration of Magnesium and Calcium in Normal Serum and Commercial Batches of Mueller-Hinton Medium

Medium* (Number of Batches Tested)	Concentration (mg/liter)†	
	Mg^{++}	Ca^{++}
M-H broth		
BBL (5)	3.0 ± 0.8 (2.0–4.7)	10.8 ± 10.4 (4.1–31.6)
Difco (5)	4.2 ± 1.0 (2.9–5.6)	15.8 ± 10.5 (8.0–35.8)
M-H agar		
BBL (6)	16.7 ± 2.9 (13.5–19.0)	50.8 ± 19.7 (32.2–86.0)
Difco (7)	26.3 ± 7.5 (9.8–32.6)	70.7 ± 16.6 (31.8–83.1)
Pfizer (10)	17.8 ± 7.5 (9.4–30.0)	46.8 ± 5.6 (41.0–63.1)
Human Serum (60)	21.7 ± 1.2	98.0 ± 2.5

SOURCE: Data adapted from L. B. Reller et al. 1974. J. Infect. Dis. *130:*456.

* M-H = Mueller-Hinton; BBL = Baltimore Biological Laboratories, Baltimore, Md.; Difco = Difco Laboratories, Detroit, Mich.; Pfizer = Pfizer Diagnostics, New York. N. Y.

† Mean ± SD (Min.–Max.).

volume of solvent required to achieve the desired concentration may be calculated by dividing the weight (μg) of active substance in the sample by the desired concentration (μg/ml). The following formula may be used:

Volume of solvent =
$$\frac{\text{Weight of sample (mg)} \times \text{activity standard (μg or IU/mg)}}{\text{Desired concentration (μg or IU/ml)}}$$

The standard powder should be weighed accurately on an analytical balance. The sample may be weighed and dissolved in the same beaker, or a weighing boat may be used and the powder washed into a large beaker with the solvent.

With most antimicrobial agents, the stock solutions can be prepared in distilled water, but to achieve solubility and to improve stability, some antimicrobics should be dissolved initially in other solvents, as listed in Table 4-3. Once dissolved in a minimum volume of solvent, most antimicrobics can be diluted further in distilled water, but with some antimicrobics, stability is improved if they are diluted in a phosphate buffer. Satisfactory phosphate buffers can be prepared as outlined in Table 4-4.

Although it is not usually necessary to sterilize stock solutions containing high concentrations of antimicrobics, the solutions may be sterilized by filtration through membrane or sintered glass filters; asbestos pads should not be used because they may absorb active substances.

Convenient volumes of the concentrated stock solutions may be distributed into individual containers that can be tightly sealed and stored at –20°C or colder. When needed, a vial may be removed from the freezer and allowed to thaw. It must be used the same day and never refrozen. Stock solutions of most antimicrobics are stable in the frozen state for at least six months, provided that the solution has not been exposed inadvertently to repeated freeze-thaw cycles, as may occur with mechanical failures of the freezer, and provided that the tubes are tightly sealed so as to minimize evaporation during storage. Appropriate quality-control procedures are essential to detection of both inactivation of the stored stock solutions and errors in their preparation.

RANGE OF CONCENTRATIONS TO BE TESTED

The actual test dilutions of antimicrobic are prepared from the stock solutions, generally as a series of doubling dilutions. The exact method by which doubling dilutions are prepared depends upon the volume of work being handled and the particular type of

Table 4-3. Solvents and Diluents for Stock Solutions of Antimicrobial Agents

Antimicrobial Agent*	Solvent	Diluent
Ampicillin	Phosphate buffer, pH 8.0, 0.1 M	Phosphate buffer, pH 6.0, 0.1 M
Carbenicillin	Water	Water
Cephalothin	Phosphate buffer, pH 6.0, 0.1 M	Water
Chloramphenicol	Ethanol	Water
Clindamycin	Water	Water
Cycloserine	Water	Water
Erythromycin	Ethanol	Water
Ethambutol	Water	Water
Flucytosine	Saline, 0.85%	Saline, 0.85%
Gentamicin	Phosphate buffer, pH 8.0, 0.1 M	Water
Isoniazid	Water	Water
Kanamycin	Phosphate buffer, pH 8, 0.1 M	Water
Nalidixic acid	NaOH, 1 N	Water
Nitrofurantoin†	Dimethylformamide	Water
Oxacillin	Water	Water
p-Aminosalicylic acid	Water	Water
Penicillin	Water	Water
Polymyxin B	Water	Water
Rifampin	Dimethylsulfoxide	Phosphate buffer, pH 7.0
Streptomycin	Water	Water
Sulfonamides	Hot water + minimal amount of 10% NaOH to dissolve	Water
Tetracycline	Water	Water
Vancomycin	Water	Water

Source: J. A. Washington and Arthur L. Barry. 1974. In *Manual of Clinical Microbiology*, 2d ed. E. H. Lennette, E. H. Spaulding and J. P. Truant (Eds.). American Society for Microbiology, Washington, D. C. p. 411.

* The dry weight of the antimicrobial agent must be multiplied by the "activity standard" provided by the manufacturer: e.g., 1 mg = 825 μg of active substance ("activity standard"); therefore, 100 mg = 82,500 μg, and 41.25 ml of solvent must be added to yield a solution with an activity of 2,000 μg/ml.

† The sodium salt is water soluble.

dilution technique being used (Chapters 5 and 6). In general, the upper limits should represent the highest concentration that could be expected *in vivo*. When one is dealing with isolates from urinary tract infections or when the drug is to be administered in massive doses, the initial concentration should be greater than that normally required. Serial dilutions should be extended below the medium

Table 4-4. Preparation of Phosphate Buffers

Chemicals (analytical grade)	g/1,000 ml Distilled Water*		
	pH 6.0	pH 7.0	pH 8.0
$K H_2 PO_4$	1.8	4.0	0.75
$K_2 HPO_4$	8.2	13.6	16.40

* Sterilize by autoclaving.

MIC for most susceptible strains of the species being tested (Table 2-2). To permit adequate control, the range of test concentrations should include the end-point of one or more standard strains (Chapter 8). Ten to 12 doubling dilutions are generally required, but the procedure may be limited to fewer dilution steps by individualizing each test system.

For routine purposes, a concentration of 128 μg or IU/ml is a satisfactory upper limit for the testing of most antimicrobics. At least 512 μg/ml should be used as the upper limit for testing nitrofurantoin and nalidixic acid and for testing *Pseudomonas aeruginosa* against carbenicillin. With the sulfonamides, the initial concentration should be at least 1,024 μg/ml.

For the sake of standardization, the final concentration of drug at each dilution step must be uniform. The antimicrobic should be diluted so as to provide doubling dilutions above and below a base line concentration of 1 μg, IU, or μ mole/ml, i.e., 16, 8, 4, 2, 1, 0.5, 0.25, and so on. This dilution schedule permits easy expression of results on a $\log_2$ scale, as indicated in Table 4-5. Such an approach simplifies statistical manipulations and avoids the spurious accuracy implied with other methods of reporting.

Table 4-5. Conversion of MIC Values to a $\log_2$ Scale

μg/ml	$\log_2$	$\log_2 + 9$
128	7	16
64	6	15
32	5	14
16	4	13
8	3	12
4	2	11
2	1	10
1	0	9
0.5	−1	8
0.25	−2	7
0.12	−3	6

STANDARDIZATION OF INOCULUM DENSITY

As with all susceptibility tests, the inoculum size is extremely critical and must be standardized as carefully as possible. In all cases, growth is selected from at least four or five isolated colonies of similar morphologic type and transferred to a nutrient broth medium. After appropriate incubation, the density of inoculum is adjusted and further diluted to give a desired number of colony-forming units (CFU), as described for the individual techniques in Chapters 5, 6, and 7. Whether stock cultures or direct clinical isolates are being tested, the colonies should be selected from a nonselective nutrient agar plate after incubation for sufficient time to obtain colonies of the size normally seen with the particular species. With most bacteria, an overnight incubation period is sufficient, but two or three days may be needed for the more slowly growing microorganisms. The nutrient broth medium should be one that is capable of supporting rapid growth of most microorganisms, i.e., soy bean casein hydrolysate (trypticase or tryptic soy broth) or brain-heart infusion broth. Almost any other broth medium may be used if it fulfills the nutritional requirements of the test organism. Supplementation with specific growth requirements may be necessary when testing nutritionally fastidious microorganisms, provided that the additives do not develop a cloudy, turbid medium. Alternatively, colonies may be suspended directly in a small volume of broth and then turbidity adjusted immediately without further incubation. The latter approach may be used to expedite the test procedure or to test nutritionally fastidious or slow-growing microorganisms or strains that fail to produce uniform turbidity when grown in a broth culture.

Adjustment of the broth cultures or direct colony suspension is accomplished in one of two ways, following the principles developed for the standard disc diffusion technique described in Chapter 14. The first and most broadly applicable procedure for standardizing the inoculum requires adjustment of turbidity by adding nutrient broth to the cell suspension to match the turbidity of a MacFarland 0.5 turbidity standard. The standard is prepared by adding 0.5 ml of 0.048 M $BaCl_2$ (1.175% w/v $BaCl_2 \cdot 2H_2O$) to 99.5 ml of 0.35 NH_2SO_4 (1% v/v). Immediately before each use, the standard must be agitated on a vortex mixer. Unless it is contained in a heat-sealed glass tube, the standard should be replaced at least once every six months. For proper turbidity adjustment, it is helpful to use a white background and contrasting black line in combination with an adequate light source. The modified Rh-typing view box (described by Stemper and Matsen[10]) facilitates the handling and reduces the time involved in standardizing cultures by this method (Fig. 4-4). Once diluted, the inoculum suspension should be allowed to stand no longer than from 20 to 30 minutes before the tests are inoculated. This approach can be used with almost any microorganism as long as the broth medium is clear and free of particles that contribute to turbidity.

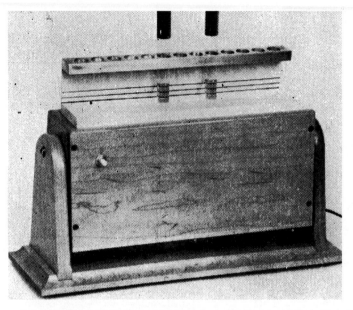

Figure 4-4. Modified Rh-typing view box for adjusting turbidity of broth cultures. (From J. E. Stemper and J. M. Matsen. 1970. Appl. Microbiol. *19:* 1015.)

The second method of adjusting the inoculum density involves the dilution of a 16-to-18 hour, 4-to-5-ml broth culture or of a 4-to-6-hour, 0.5-ml broth culture according to a predetermined schedule. This approach is limited to rapid growing *Enterobacteraciae, Staphylcoccus aureus*, enterococci, and *Pseudomonas aeruginosa*, since it depends upon the capacity of the microorganism to reach the stationary phase of growth rapidly. At that time a maximum cell concentration of about 1×10^9 CFU/ml is reached and maintained for several hours and thus further adjustment of turbidity is not required. A 1:10 dilution of such stationary phase broth cultures generally yields inocula that are comparable to those obtained by matching a MacFarland 0.5 standard (Table 4-6).

With either method of adjusting the inoculum, the cell suspension is further diluted, before inoculation of the broth or agar

Table 4-6. CFU/ml Achieved with Three Methods for Standardizing the Inoculum for Antimicrobic Susceptibility Tests

Control Strain Method of Adjustment	Mean (± S.E) (N = 28* or N = 24*)	Min.–Max. of Daily Estimates
E. coli (ATCC 25922)		
BaSO₄ Standard	$7.8\ (\pm 0.62) \times 10^7$	1.1×10^7–1.2×10^9
5 hr., 0.5 ml BHI (1:10)	$1.9\ (\pm 0.06) \times 10^8$	1.6×10^8–2.2×10^8
18 hr., 5 ml BHI (1:10)	$1.6\ (\pm 0.08) \times 10^8$	9.3×10^7–2.2×10^8
P. aeruginosa (ATCC 27853)		
BaSO₄ Standard	$1.2\ (\pm 0.10) \times 10^8$	6.5×10^8–2.2×10^9
5 hr., 0.5 ml BHI (1:10)	$2.2\ (\pm 0.15) \times 10^8$	9.2×10^7–3.4×10^8
18 hr., 5 ml BHI (1:10)	$1.2\ (\pm 0.09) \times 10^8$	5.6×10^7–2.0×10^8
S. aureus (ATCC 25923)		
BaSO₄ Standard	$1.7\ (\pm 0.11) \times 10^7$	1.5×10^7–2.0×10^7
5 hr., 0.5 ml BHI (1:10)	$7.9\ (\pm 0.89) \times 10^7$	1.9×10^7–8.1×10^7
18 hr., 5 ml BHI (1:10)	$9.2\ (\pm 0.71) \times 10^7$	2.4×10^7–6.6×10^7
Enterococcus (CDC 57657)		
BaSO₄ Standard	$6.7\ (\pm 0.28) \times 10^7$	4.8×10^7–7.9×10^7
5 hr., 0.5 ml BHI (1:10)	$2.0\ (\pm 0.07) \times 10^8$	8.7×10^7–2.2×10^8
18 hr., 5 ml BHI (1:10)	$2.6\ (\pm 0.12) \times 10^8$	1.1×10^8–2.0×10^8

SOURCE: A. L. Barry and R. A. Lasner. Unpublished data.

* Data for each method based on seven daily quadruplicate plate counts for both gram-negative bacilli (N = 28) or six daily quadruplicate plate counts for both gram-positive strains (N = 24).

media. The actual volume applied to the antimicrobic-containing medium depends upon the technique being used, and thus the inoculum is best expressed as the absolute number of CFU delivered rather than the concentration (CFU/ml) in the suspension used to inoculate the plates or tubes. For example, if an inoculum suspension is standardized to contain 10^5 CFU/ml and then broth dilution and agar dilution tests are both inoculated to compare the two methods, each agar plate receives approximately 0.002 ml, or 200 CFU per spot, whereas the broth tubes each contain 1 ml of inoculum plus an equal volume of antimicrobic-containing broth, or 50,000 CFU/ml. If a microdilution tray is inoculated with 50 μl drops of the same suspension, each receives 2,500 CFU in 0.1 ml (25,000 CFU/ml).

REFERENCES

1. Barry, A. L. 1974. The agar overlay technique for disc susceptibility testing. In *Current Techniques for Antibiotic Susceptibility Testing*. A. Balows (Ed.). Charles C Thomas, Springfield, Ill. pp. 17-25.
2. Ericsson, H. M., and J. C. Sherris. 1971. Antibiotic sensitivity testing. Report of an international collaborative study. Acta Pathol. Microbiol. Scand. Sect. B, Suppl. 217.
3. Garrod, L. P., and P. M. Waterworth. 1969. Effect of medium composition on the apparent sensitivity of *Pseudomonas aeruginosa* to gentamicin. J. Clin. Pathol. *22:* 534-538.
4. Hoeprich, P. D., A. L. Barry, and G. D. Fay. 1971. Synthetic medium for susceptibility testing. Antimicrob. Agents Chemother.1970. pp. 494-497.
5. Mueller, H. H., and J. Hinton. 1941. A protein-free medium for primary isolation of the gonococcus and meningococcus. Proc. Soc. Exp. Biol. Med. *48:*330-333.
6. Reller, L. B., F. D. Schoenknecht, M. A. Kenny, and J. C. Sherris. 1974. Antibiotic susceptibility testing of *Pseudomonas aeruginosa*: Selection of a control strain and criteria for magnesium and calcium content of media. J. Infect. Dis. *130:* 454-463.
7. Rosenblatt, J. E., and F. Schoenknecht. 1972. Effect of several components of anaerobic incubation on antibiotic susceptibility test results. Antimicrob. Agents Chemother. *1:* 433-440.
8. Ryan, A. R., G. M. Needham, C. L. Dunsmoor, and J. C. Sherris. 1970. Stability of antibiotics and chemotherapeutics in agar plates. Appl. Microbiol. *20:* 447-451.
9. Steers, E., E. L. Foltz, and B. S. Graves. 1959. An inocula replicating apparatus for routine testing of bacterial susceptibility to antibiotics. Antibiot. Chemother. *9:* 307-311.
10. Stemper, J. E., and J. M. Matsen. 1970. Device for turbidity standardization of cultures for antibiotic sensitivity testing. Appl. Microbiol. *19:* 1015-1016.
11. Vera, H. D., and M. Dumoff. 1974. Culture media. In *Manual of Clinical Microbiology*. 2nd ed. E. H. Lennette, E. H. Spaulding, and J. P. Truant (Eds.). American Society for Microbiology, Washington, D. C. pp. 879-929.
12. Washington, J. A. 1971. The agar-diffusion method. In *Antimicrobial Susceptibility Testing*. T. L. Gavan, H. W. McFadden, and E. Cheattle (Eds.). American Society of Clinical Pathologists Inc., Chicago, Ill. pp. 127-141.
13. Washington, J. A., E. Warren, C. T. Dolan, and A. G. Karlson. 1974. Tests to determine the activity of antimicrobial agents. In *Laboratory Procedures in Clinical Microbiology*. J. A. Washington (Ed.). Little, Brown, Boston. pp. 281-340.
14. Washington, J. A., E. Warren, and A. G. Karlson. 1973. Stability of barium sulfate turbidity standards. Appl. Microbiol. *24:* 1013.

Chapter 5

AGAR DILUTION TECHNIQUES

Agar dilution susceptibility tests are performed by incorporating the antimicrobial agent into an agar medium just before it is poured onto a petri plate. With an inoculum-replicating apparatus, as many as 36 strains can be spot-inoculated simultaneously onto each of a series of petri plates containing varying concentrations of antimicrobic. Agar dilution techniques have three major advantages over broth dilution techniques: (1) the capacity to test a fairly large number of strains at the same time, (2) the ability to detect microbial heterogeneity or contamination because of the nature of bacterial growth on the surface of an agar plate as compared to that in a broth medium, and (3) the ability to supplement the medium with whole blood or blood products so as to permit testing of some of the nutritionally fastidious microorganisms that cannot be tested satisfactorily in a clear broth medium.

PREPARATION OF TEST PLATES

Selection of Agar Medium. Mueller-Hinton agar is recommended for testing most rapid-growing bacterial pathogens, but with some microorganisms additional supplements are needed to obtain sufficiently rapid growth. Satisfactory results have been reported when this medium is supplemented with "chocolatized" blood, with 5% (v/v) laked blood (lysed by repeated freeze-thaw cycles), or with 5% (v/v) peptic digest of blood. Addition of blood or blood products has little effect on antimicrobic activity, except in the case of highly protein–bound drugs, such as novobiocin. The activity of the sulfonamides is partially antagonized by all blood products, but the results are markedly improved by the addition of laked horse blood, probably because of a high concentration of thymidinase. Defibrinated blood should be added for testing streptococci; "chocolatized" blood or peptic digest of blood may be added for testing *Hemophilus* sp. or *Neisseria gonorrhoeae*; and laked blood is recommended by some authors for testing the sulfonamides. When testing *Staphylococcus aureus* against the methicillin family of drugs, 5% NaCl (w/v) may be added to the Mueller-Hinton agar for earlier detection of resistant variants. Unsupplemented Mueller-Hinton agar is satisfactory for testing most other aerobic or facultatively anaerobic bacterial pathogens, including *N. meningitidis*.

Preparation of Antimicrobic Plates. Dilutions of the antimicrobial agent are prepared in sterile distilled water at a concentration ten times that desired in the final test. The dilution scheme outlined in Table 5-1 is recommended because it is relatively simple to perform, economical of pipettes (because only one pipette need be used for each block of three dilutions), and because the method is not subject to the same cumulative error inherent in traditional serial dilution methods. The range of dilutions shown in Table 5-1 are only illustrative; the dilution series may begin or end at any point desired. The total volumes actually prepared can be adjusted according to the number of microorganisms to be tested. For routine clinical laboratory application, it may be necessary to limit the dilution series to only three to four plates per antimicrobic, using dilution steps that deviate from the standard doubling dilution scheme. An example of such a shortened series of dilutions is outlined in Table 5-2.

The agar medium is prepared in screw-cap bottles, flasks, or tubes and allowed to cool from 45° to 50°C in a water bath. Sufficient volumes are prepared to fill each 9-cm petri plate with from 20 to 25 ml of agar. The diluted antimicrobic solutions are added to the melted and cooled medium in a ratio of one part antimicrobic to nine parts of medium (2 ml of drug to 18 ml of agar for each petri plate). The medium is then mixed by gently inverting the tube or flask several times, and the content is poured onto the appropriate number of petri plates. If necessary, blood or blood products may be added immediately after the antimicrobic and before mixing and pouring. The plates are then set aside on a flat horizontal surface

Table 5-1. A Dilution Scheme for Preparation of Agar Dilution Susceptibility Plates

Volume* of Drug Solution and Concentration (μg or IU/ml)		Volume* of Sterile Water		Concentration (μg or IU/ml)		
				Intermediate	Final†	Log_2
6.4 ml	2,000 μg/ml stock	+ 3.6 ml	=	1,280 μg/ml	128	7
2 vols	1,280 μg/ml (above)	+ 2 vols	=	640 μg/ml	64	6
1 vol	1,280 μg/ml (above)	+ 3 vols	=	320 μg/ml	32	5
1 vol	1,280 μg/ml (above)	+ 7 vols	=	160 μg/ml	16	4
2 vols	160 μg/ml (above)	+ 2 vols	=	80 μg/ml	8	3
1 vol	160 μg/ml (above)	+ 3 vols	=	40 μg/ml	4	2
1 vol	160 μg/ml (above)	+ 7 vols	=	20 μg/ml	2	1
2 vols	20 μg/ml (above)	+ 2 vols	=	10 μg/ml	1	0
1 vol	20 μg/ml (above)	+ 3 vols	=	5 μg/ml	0.5	−1
1 vol	20 μg/ml (above)	+ 7 vols	=	2.5 μg/ml	0.25	−2
etc.				etc.		etc.

* Any multiple of the volumes in the table may be used, according to the number of petri plates to be prepared for each drug concentration. At least 2 ml of drug and 18 ml of agar will be needed for each 9-cm petri plate.

† The final concentration is based on the addition of 1 part of drug solution to 9 parts of melted and cooled (50°C) agar medium.

Table 5-2. An Abbreviated Dilution Schedule for Screening Bacterial Isolates by the Agar Dilution Technique

	Concentrations (μg/ml)											
Antimicrobial	0.01	0.1	0.5	1.0	3.0	5.0	10.0	20.0	50.0	100	200	300
Ampicillin	–	–	–	X	–	X	X	X	–	X	X	–
Carbenicillin	–	–	–	–	–	–	–	–	X	X	X	–
Cephalothin	–	–	–	X	–	X	X	X	–	X	–	–
Chloramphenicol	–	–	–	–	–	X	X	X	–	–	–	–
Clindamycin	–	–	–	X	–	X	–	–	–	–	–	–
Erythromycin	–	X	–	X	–	X	–	–	–	–	–	–
Gentamicin	–	–	–	X	X	X	X	–	–	–	–	–
Kanamycin	–	–	–	X	–	X	X	–	–	X	–	–
Nalidixic acid	–	–	–	–	–	–	X	–	X	X	–	–
Nitrofurantoin	–	–	–	–	–	–	–	–	X	X	–	X
Oxacillin	–	–	–	X	–	X	X	–	–	–	–	–
Penicillin	–	X	X	X	–	X	–	–	–	–	–	–
Polymyxin B	–	–	–	X	–	X	X	–	–	–	–	–
Tetracycline	–	–	–	X	–	X	X	–	–	–	–	–
Vancomycin	–	X	–	X	–	X	–	–	–	–	–	–

SOURCE: J. A. Washington, E. Warren, C. T. Dolan, and A. G. Karlson. 1974. In *Laboratory Procedures in Clinical Microbiology*. J. A. Washington (Ed.). Little, Brown, Boston. p. 288.

and allowed to harden undisturbed. At least one control plate, containing Mueller-Hinton agar without antimicrobic, is prepared for every series of dilutions. For reference work, the plates should be used within 24 hours of preparation (they should be held in the refrigerator if not used on the day of preparation). For most other purposes, the antimicrobic-containing plates can be refrigerated in sealed plastic bags for at least one week without a significant loss of antimicrobic activity. Many drugs can be stored for as long as four weeks without deterioration, provided that evaporation is minimized by carefully sealing the plates in plastic bags. The plastic bags within which most plastic petri plates are distributed are ideally suited for storage of antimicrobic-containing plates. Quality-control procedures must be utilized to detect any loss of activity during storage, to detect contamination (especially if blood products have been added), and to detect any loss of nutritive capacity during preparation and storage. Since agar media stored in this way often contain a considerable amount of surface moisture, the plates must be allowed to dry in a 35°C incubator with lids ajar just before they are to be inoculated.

TEST PROCEDURES

Standardization of Inoculum. For each strain to be tested, broth cultures are initiated by inoculating growth from four or five freshly isolated colonies into the appropriate nutrient broth. After a sufficient period of incubation, the inoculum is standardized according to the methods outlined in Chapter 4. That is, either (1) adjust the turbidity of a four-to-six-hour broth culture to match that of a MacFarland 0.5 turbidity standard, (2) dilute a four-to-six-hour, 0.5-ml broth culture according to a predetermined dilution scheme, or (3) dilute a 16-to-18-hour, 4-ml broth culture according to the same predetermined schedule. Simple dilution of an overnight broth culture is often the most convenient method for handling large surveys, but the other two methods described above are generally more applicable to the routine clinical laboratory, where time is of the essence. The last two methods, which depend upon the microorganisms reaching a stationary phase of growth, are applicable only to tests with rapid-growing *Enterobacteriaceae*, *Staphylococcus aureus*, most enterococci, and *Pseudomonas* sp. Microorganisms that belong to other genera or strains that are unusually slow-growing or fail to produce uniformly turbid growth in broth should be standardized by adjusting to match a turbidity standard. With nutritionally fastidious microorganisms that fail to grow in a clear broth medium, the inoculum may be standardized by suspending freshly isolated colonies directly in a small volume of saline solution and then adjusting turbidity immediately, without further incubation.

Inoculation of Agar Plates. The standardized suspension prepared as described above is then diluted further in saline so as to yield a suspension containing about 5×10^6 viable cells per ml (a 1:20 dilution of a suspension adjusted to match that of a MacFarland standard or a 1:200 dilution of a stationary-phase broth culture). This suspension is then spotted onto the previously dried surface of each antimicrobic-containing plate. The inoculum is applied as a spot that covers the circle of about 5 to 8 mm in diameter. The spot is then allowed to dry without spreading, and thus many strains can be tested on the same plate. The inoculum may be applied with a loop calibrated to deliver 0.001 ml or with an inoculum replicator, such as that depicted in Figure 5-1. The later has been found to be capable of delivering about 0.001 to 0.003 ml with each prong. Consequently, each spot should contain about 1×10^4 viable cells in a circle from 5 to 8 mm in diameter.

If an inoculum-replicating apparatus is used, a portion of the diluted cell suspension is transferred to the appropriate well in the seed plate and then the inocula are picked up and gently transferred to the agar surface, being careful to avoid splashing. Control plates without antimicrobic should be inoculated last to insure that viable microorganisms were present throughout the procedure. Inoculation of the test plates should be completed within 30 minutes of adjustment of the turbidity of the first strain. An aluminum replicating device,[11] such as that pictured in Figure 5-1, is available

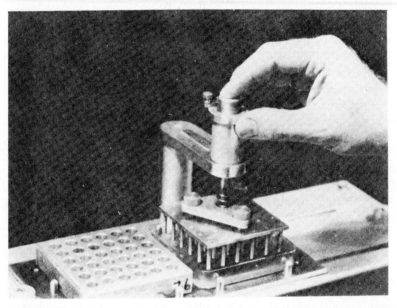

Figure 5-1. Steers' inoculum-replicating apparatus[11] with seed plate containing 36 reservoirs at left. Plate with medium containing antibiotic is being inoculated. (From J. A. Washington, E. Warren, C. T. Dolan, and A. G. Karlson. 1974. In *Laboratory Procedures in Clinical Microbiology*. J. A. Washington (Ed.). Little, Brown, Boston. p. 287.)

commercially.* Stainless-steel heads are easier to clean and less subject to corrosion. Many investigators find a hand-held version of this inoculum replicator to be just as convenient and efficient as that shown in Figure 5-1. After use, the seed plates and inoculating prongs are soaked overnight in 70% ethyl alcohol, scrubbed clean with a brush, and wrapped in a cloth towel. This pack is then sterilized by autoclaving before use.

Special precautions must be taken in testing microorganisms that produce swarming or spreading growth, e.g., *Proteus mirabilis* and

* Melrose Machine Shop (176 Fairview Road, Woodlyn, Pa. 19094).

P. vulgaris. Each inoculated spot must be isolated from the others with a mechanical barrier. A glass cylinder approximately 12 mm in diameter may be pressed firmly onto the agar and left in place during incubation. Alternatively, the inoculated spot may be isolated by removing strips of agar between each inoculated area. Attempts to inhibit swarming by increasing the concentration of agar or by decreasing salt concentrations should be avoided since the activity of some antimicrobics will be affected.

Incubation of Test Plates. The inoculated plates are allowed to stand undisturbed until the spots of inoculum have all been absorbed completely. The plates are inverted and allowed to incubate at 35°C for 16 to 20 hours. Whenever possible, incubation under an increased CO_2 atmosphere should be avoided because of the resulting increase in surface pH, which has an adverse affect on the activity of many antimicrobic agents. However, those microorganisms that fail to grow in the absence of an increased CO_2 atmosphere may be tested, provided that adequate controls are included and appropriate precautions are taken in interpretation of the results. Each time such microorganisms are to be tested, one or more control strains should be tested in duplicate—one set of plates incubated aerobically and another under increased CO_2. These controls indicate the direction and extent to which the CO_2 atmosphere affects the MICs with the drug under study and thus provide a clue as to the extent to which one can rely upon the MICs obtained with the capnophilic microorganism.

Reading Test Results. After from 16 to 18 hours of incubation, the agar dilution plates are examined for growth. First, the control plate without antimicrobic is checked to be sure that each test strain was capable of providing adequate growth. The remaining plates are then examined to determine the minimal concentration of drug required for inhibition of growth. In reading the end-points, a faint haze of growth or growth of a single colony is disregarded, whereas a definite dense film of growth or more than one colony is considered evidence that the antimicrobic failed to inhibit growth adequately at that concentration. If several isolated colonies are found within a spot of otherwise inhibited growth, the purity of the strain should be checked, especially if isolated colonies are found to extend through two or more doubling dilutions beyond an obvious end-point. One important advantage to the agar dilution technique is its ability to detect mixed cultures or contamination, whereas the broth dilution technique only expresses the MIC of the most resistant member of the bacterial population.

When testing microorganisms that fail to grow adequately within 16 to 18 hours, the plates may be re-incubated and read after 48 hours of incubation. For such tests, one or more control strains should be included and the MICs recorded after overnight incubation and again after 48 hours. If the end-points for the controls do not change, it should be safe to assume that the drug has not deteriorated significantly and thus the MICs for the slow-growing microorganisms can be reported.

ANTIMICROBIC SUSCEPTIBILITY OF
Neisseria gonorrhoeae

This species remains uniformly susceptible to benzylpenicillin at concentrations obtained in the blood of patients treated with doses currently recommended for chemotherapy of gonorrhea. However, over the years there has been a gradual increase in the amount of penicillin required to inhibit growth of some strains: MICs of from 2 to 4 IU/ml have been reported,[8] and increasingly larger doses are being recommended. *In vitro* susceptibility to benzylpenicillin has not been found to correlate well with the responsiveness or nonresponsiveness of the individual patient to penicillin therapy, and thus routine susceptibility testing of *N. gonorrhoeae* isolates is not indicated clinically. However, clinical centers with the technical capability should continue to monitor the level of susceptibility among clinical isolates to maintain surveillance of the changing situation in regard to penicillin susceptibility and susceptibility to other antimicrobics. For such epidemiologic and research purposes, *in vitro* susceptibility tests can be performed reliably with the agar dilution technique, modified slightly to permit growth of *N. gonorrhoeae*.

Clinical isolates may be held at –60°C or lower until the tests can be performed conveniently. After a pure culture is obtained, several colonies are suspended in a small volume of trypticase soy broth (without glucose), with 15% (v/v) glycerol added and the resulting dense suspension placed directly into the freezer. Just before testing, the isolates are allowed to thaw and are transferred to freshly prepared chocolate agar plates. After 48 hours of incubation in a moist chamber with an increased CO_2 atmosphere, several isolated colonies are selected for testing.

At least four or five colonies are suspended in trypticase soy broth and then adjusted by adding broth until the turbidity matches that of a MacFarland 0.5 standard. This suspension should contain 10^7 to 10^8 CFU/ml, and a 1:20 dilution in broth is spotted directly onto the antimicrobic plates as described for other agar dilution tests. Antimicrobic dilutions are prepared and incorporated into gonococcal medium base (Bacto-GC medium, Difco) enriched with 1% (w/v) hemoglobin and 1% (v/v) Isovitalex (BBL) or supplement C (Difco). The test plates should be inoculated within 48 hours of preparation. The agar surface is dried at 35°C with lids ajar just before inoculation.

The inoculated plates are inverted and allowed to incubate at 35°C in a moist chamber with an increased CO_2 atmosphere. After 24 hours of incubation, the plates are examined and the MIC recorded as described for other agar dilution tests. If the control fails to demonstrate sufficient growth, the test may be re-incubated and examined again after 48 hours. Decreased susceptibility among strains requiring 48 hours for growth may be reported only if control strains showed no significant differences between 24-hour and 48-hour MICs.

With each batch of tests, a control strain of *Neisseria gonorrhoeae* of known susceptibility and a stock culture of *Sarcina lutea* should be included to provide a control of technical procedures. The density of inoculum is an important variable, and randomly selected samples of the test strains should be checked by further diluting the adjusted cell suspension 1:50 and then streaking a chocolate agar plate with a 0.001 ml calibrated loopful of this dilution. This should produce from 10 to 100 colonies. Strains that demonstrate decreased susceptibility should not be reported unless the inoculum density has been checked. At times, that requires repeated testing of strains showing slightly elevated MIC's but it insures reliability of test results.

ANTIMICROBIC SUSCEPTIBILITY OF
Hemophilus influenzae

Clinically significant isolates of *H. influenzae* are virtually all susceptible to ampicillin or chloramphenicol. Ampicillin-resistant strains of *H. influenzae* have been recovered recently from the spinal fluid of patients with meningitis,[5] and for that reason significant isolates should be tested against ampicillin as soon as they are recovered. Such routine tests are fraught with difficulty, especially when the disc diffusion technique is utilized. Susceptible strains often appear to be resistant because of technical problems. When resistance has been detected, it is more likely to represent a technical problem rather than "true" ampicillin resistance. As an alternative to routinely testing individual isolates as they are recovered, strains may be stored for short periods of time and later tested under carefully standardized conditions with appropriate controls. As long as resistance remains a very infrequent occurrence, such monitoring of susceptibility with an antimicrobic dilution technique might be the best, most practical method for obtaining and maintaining controlled test conditions.

Methods for testing of *H. influenzae* have not yet been standardized sufficiently well to support the description of a routine testing procedure. Experienced investigators have not yet been able to agree upon a standard method for performing antimicrobic dilution tests with *H. influenzae.* Some prefer broth dilution techniques, other prefer agar dilution methods; in all cases the medium must be supplemented in order to support growth of the test organisms. Additives that have been recommended are: (1) chocolate agar (either GC medium or Mueller-Hinton agar base with heated blood or with hemoglobin and a source of DPN), (2) 5% (v/v) peptic digest of blood, (3) yeast autolysate (supplement C), (4) unlysed rabbit blood or horse blood plus 1% Isovitalex (BBL), (5) laked horse blood, or (6) Leventhal's medium.

The number of viable cells in the inoculum is particularly critical when testing *H. influenzae* against the penicillins, especially with the agar dilution technique. The greater the inoculum the greater the concentration of antimicrobic required for inhibition of growth. When a large inoculum is used, a significant number of susceptible strains display penicillin G and ampicillin MICs that exceed the concentration ordinarily obtained during chemotherapy.[6] With these drugs, the end-points are rather poorly defined, and a marked decrease in the amount of growth is seen over several dilution steps below the MIC. When the inoculum is reduced, the end-points are better defined and the susceptible strains all have MICs well below obtainable blood levels. The inoculum density seems to be more critical with the agar dilution technique than with the broth dilution method.[6]

Until a standard method is developed for testing *H. influenzae* susceptibility to ampicillin, the following procedure can be recommended as an interim agar dilution method for monitoring susceptibility of clinical isolates:

The day before testing, the isolates are transferred to freshly prepared chocolate agar plates. After overnight incubation in an increased CO_2 atmosphere, the plates are examined and from five to ten colonies selected for testing. The colonies are suspended in a small volume of trypticase soy broth and then adjusted with the same soy broth medium until the turbidity matches that of a MacFarland 0.5 standard. This suspension should contain about 10^8 CFU/ml, and a 1:100 dilution is then prepared in trypticase soy broth. This diluted suspension should contain about 10^6 CFU/ml and thus, when spotted onto the antimicrobic plates, each spot should contain approximately 1,000 to 3,000 CFU. The actual inoculum density obtained should be checked by testing randomly selected samples of the test strains within each test series. This may be accomplished by preparing a 1:10 dilution of the inoculum and then streaking an antimicrobic-free control plate with a 0.001-ml calibrated loopful of this suspension. An adequately prepared inoculum should produce from 10 to 100 colonies. Strains with increased resistance to ampicillin should be retested if this control indicates an excessively heavy inoculum.

Antimicrobic dilutions are prepared and incorporated into Mueller-Hinton agar supplemented with 5% (v/v) Fildes peptic digest of blood. To prepare the latter supplement, thoroughly mix in a screw-cap flask: 150 ml of 0.85% NaCl, 6 ml of concentrated HCl, 50 ml of defibrinated sheep blood, and 1 g of granular pepsin. Place the mixture in a 55°C water bath, shaking it occasionally during the first two hours and then leaving it in the water bath overnight. After from 16 to 18 hours at 55°C, add about 6 ml of 5 N NaOH until the pH is 7 or slightly less. Aseptically divide the digested blood into convenient aliquots in sterile bottles or tubes and store several weeks in the refrigerator or up to one year in the freezer. Before use, warm the peptic digest gently and add it to the sterilized agar base in a ratio of 5 ml of peptic digest to 100 ml of agar medium.

For ampicillin or penicillin G, the final concentration of drug should range from 32 to 0.06 μg/ml, and for chloramphenicol and tetracycline concentrations should range from 64 to 0.12 μg/ml. For each series of tests prepare a sufficient number of antimicrobic-free control plates to provide growth controls and to permit a check on the inoculum density of a significant sample of the strains being tested.

The MIC is determined after from 16 to 18 hours at 35°C, as described for other agar dilution tests. With this system, susceptible strains are usually inhibited by 1 μg/ml or less, except when an unusually heavy inoculum has been achieved. Ampicillin-resistant strains should require at least 8 μg/ml for inhibition.

ANTIMICROBIC SUSCEPTIBILITY OF ANAEROBIC BACTERIA

An increasing awareness of anaerobic microorganisms and their role in infectious diseases has placed new demands upon the clinical laboratory. Once anaerobes have been recovered from a clinical specimen, attention is drawn to the question of selecting the most appropriate chemotherapy and the laboratory is often requested to perform susceptibility tests with each individual isolate that has been recovered. Such tests are fraught with problems related to technique and interpretation of results. Since the majority of anaerobic infections involve several microorganisms (even though only one species may be recovered), the susceptibility of individual isolates may or may not be significant. There is good reason to believe that antimicrobic therapy does not necessarily need to ir-radicate all species within an abscess since some are simple commensals that will be eliminated once the infectious process has been brought under control and others are symbionts incapable of surviving alone.[1,2,13]

Isolation of anaerobes and performance of susceptibility tests on individual isolates is necessarily a slow process. It may require an average of from five to ten days. For that reason, initial chemotherapy of suspected anaerobic infections is usually deter-mined empirically after the appropriate specimens have been collected and processed. This is possible because there is generally a high level of predictability of antimicrobic susceptibility among commonly encountered anaerobic bacteria. However, those centers with the technical capacity should continue to monitor the situation among clinical isolates. By tabulating and compiling reports of sus-ceptibility tests with different anaerobes, the empirical basis of chemotherapy can reflect any changes in susceptibility patterns that may appear within the community. To permit a comparison of data collected in different laboratories, a single standardized method must be adopted. Unfortunately, such a standardized method has not yet been agreed upon. Until such a standardized technique is described, the following agar dilution method may be recommended as an interim technique.

Individual isolates may be stored at −60°C or lower until the tests can be performed conveniently. Once recovered in pure culture, growth is scraped from a 48-hour agar plate culture and suspended in 10% skim milk (20% dehydrated skim milk plus an equal volume of cell suspension). Just before testing, the isolates are allowed to thaw and transferred to freshly prepared blood agar plates, and after 48 hours of incubation under anaerobic conditions each isolate is checked for purity and viability. Aerobic blood agar plates are also inoculated to rule out the possibility of contamination with aerobes.

Portions of four or five isolated colonies with similar morphology are transferred to a tube of modified thioglycollate medium without indicator (BBL-135C). This medium is enriched with hemin, 5 μg/ml, and vitamin K_1, 0.1 μg/ml (added prior to sterilization), and

NaHCO$_3$, 1 mg/ml (added aseptically after autoclaving). This medium should be stored at room temperature and used within two weeks of preparation. After overnight incubation, or as soon as visible turbidity appears, the broth cultures are diluted so as to obtain a turbidity that matches that of a MacFarland 0.5 standard. This suspension is then used, without further dilution, for inoculation of the antimicrobic-containing plates (employing an inoculum replicator, as described for other agar dilution tests). Each plate should receive approximately 10^5 CFU/spot.

On the day of the test, dilutions of the stock antimicrobic solutions are prepared and incorporated into agar plates as described previously. The agar medium consists of Brucella agar (Pfizer) containing Vitamin K$_1$, 10 μg/ml added just before autoclaving and further supplemented with 5% (v/v) laked defibrinated sheep blood (lysed by repeated freeze-thaw cycles).

The plates are spot-inoculated with an inoculum replicator or a calibrated loop, as for other agar dilution tests. The plates are then allowed to incubate 48 hours at 35°C in a Gas-Pak (BBL) jar. One control plate is incubated anaerobically to serve as growth control, and the other is incubated aerobically to detect aerobic contamination. The MIC of each strain is then determined as the lowest concentration of drug yielding no growth, one or two discreet colonies, or a fine barely visible haze of growth—provided that the growth controls indicate viability under these conditions. A stock control strain should be maintained and included in each series of tests in order to insure consistency of results.

For clinical application, the antimicrobics that generally need to be tested include penicillin, tetracycline, clindamycin, and chloramphenicol. Metronidazole susceptibility may be indicated if this agent is approved for therapy of anaerobic infections. Table 5-3 depicts the general level of susceptibility observed with clinical isolates of anaerobic bacteria tested by a broth dilution technique.[17]

A disc elution test was described in 1973 by Wilkins and Thiel.[19] This appears to be a reliable, simple method for determining susceptibility of individual isolates. Commercial antibiotic discs are added anaerobically to tubes of prereduced brain-heart infusion broth so as to achieve concentrations approaching that attainable in the blood. The tubes are then inoculated and incubated overnight. Susceptibility is then attributed to an anaerobe that produces a turbidity no greater than 50% of that of the control culture. As originally described, this anaerobic disc-broth technique provides only qualitative information but it could be adapted to provide a quantitative estimate of susceptibility. Further experience with

Table 5-3. Broth Dilution MICs with *Bacteroidaceae* Isolated from Blood Cultures, 1970 to 1972

Antimicrobic Species	Number of Strains	Cumulative % Inhibited by Increasing Concentration (µg/ml)										
		0.1	0.2	0.4	0.8	1.6	3.1	6.2	12.5	25	50	100
Penicillin G												
B. fragilis	159					1	2	5	13	23	45	62	75
Other*	16	25	44	44	63	69	69	75	75	94	94	94
Erythromycin												
B. fragilis	159	2	4	16	39	60	73	84	92	94		
Other	16	6	18	24	30	54	54	62	70	81		
Tetracycline												
B. fragilis	159	5	9	21	26	30	33	38	54	72	95	97
Other	15	26	53	73	87	100						
Clindamycin												
B. fragilis	119	50	63	78	87	95	97	99	100			
Other	14	31	70	75	75	81	81	81	88			
Chloramphenicol												
B. fragilis	159	1	1	2	2	4	20	65	90	96	100	
Other	16	6	6	12	18	44	85	75	88		94	
Metronidazole												
B. fragilis	21					33	57	95	100			
Other	4	25	50	50	100							

SOURCE: J. A. Washington, W. J. Martin, and P. E. Hermans. 1974. In *Anaerobic Bacteria: Role in Disease.* A. Balows, R. M. DeHaan, V. R. Dowell, and L. B. Guze (Eds.). Charles C Thomas, Springfield, Ill. p. 489.

* Includes: 8 *Fusobacterium nucleatum*, 1 *F. varium*, 2 *Bacteroides* (CDC group F₁, 1 *B. incommunis*, 1 *B. oralis*, 2 *B. melaninogenicus* and 1 *Bacteroides* sp.

this procedure will be needed before a recommendation can be made for its general use. The agar dilution technique is generally considered the most practical and most reliable reference method for monitoring susceptibility among clinical isolates of anaerobic bacteria. An agar diffusion technique is described in the following section.

DETECTION OF METHICILLIN-RESISTANT
Staphylococcus aureus

Strains of *S. aureus* that are resistant to methicillin and related drugs often display a marked heterogeneity, i.e., a small proportion of individual cells are resistant while the majority of cells are fully susceptible. Unless special precautions are taken, the resistant por-

tion of the population might not be detected. The following procedures have been suggested as an aid in detection:

1. Reduction of incubator temperatures (30°C)
2. Addition of 5% (w/v) NaCl to the test medium
3. Extension of incubation time to 48 hours
4. Use of a very large inoculum

The standardized agar dilution technique is generally satisfactory if the medium is stabilized osmotically with NaCl (5%) and if
the temperature is held at 35°C or less. Incubation at 37°C rather
than 35°C severely compromises the ability of the test to detect
methicillin resistance. With one or more of the above modifications
of the standard agar dilution technique, resistant strains of *S. aureus* should grow in the presence of 8 μg methicillin per ml or 4 μg
oxacillin or nafcillin per ml, whereas susceptible strains will be
inhibited by that concentration.

In most medical centers across the United States, methicillin-
resistant strains of *S. aureus* are rarely seen. In practice, reports of
methicillin-resistant *S. aureus* often represent *S. epidermidis* that
have been misidentified for some reason. Methicillin resistance
among strains of *S. epidermidis* is not uncommon, and mixtures of
resistant *S. epidermidis* and susceptible *S. aureus* are often found
in clinical material. The identification of resistant colonies growing
on antimicrobic-containing plates should be confirmed before
being reported as methicillin-resistant *S. aureus*.

REFERENCES

1. Gorbach, S. L., and J. G. Bartlett. 1974. Anaerobic infections. N. Eng. J. Med. (3 pts.) *290*: 1177-1184; 1237-1245; 1289-1294.
2. Gorbach, S. L., and J. G. Bartlett. 1974. Anaerobic infections: Old myths and new realities. J. Infect. Dis. *130*: 307-310.
3. Hewitt, J. H., A. W. Coe, and M. T. Parker. 1969. The detection of methicillin resistance in *Staphylococcus aureus*. J. Med. Microbiol. *2*: 443-456.
4. Hollander, H. O., G. Laurell, and K. Dornbusch. 1969. Determination of methicillin resistance of *Staphylococcus aureus*. Scand. J. Infect. Dis. *1*: 169-174.
5. Knapp, R. A., M. S. Dickerson, T. Peele, and C. L. Nayfield. 1974. Ampicillin-resistant *Hemophilus influenzae* meningitis. Morbidity and Mortality Weekly Report *23*: 202-207.
6. McLinn, S. E., J. D. Nelson, and K. C. Haltalin. 1970. Antimicrobial susceptibility of *Hemophilus influenzae*. Pediatrics *45*: 827-838.
7. Reyn, A., M. W. Bentzon, J. D. Thayer, and A. E. Wilkinson. 1965. Results of comparative experiments using different methods for determining the sensitivity of *Neisseria gonorrhoeae* to penicillin G. Bull. WHO *32*: 477-502.
8. Ronald, A. R., J. Eby, and J. C. Sherris. 1968. Susceptibility of *Neisseria gonorrhoeae* to penicillin and tetracycline. Antimicrob. Agents Chemother. *8*: 431-434.
9. Rosenblatt, J. E., and F. Schoenknecht. 1972. Effect of several components of anaerobic incubation on antibiotic susceptibility test results. Antimicrob. Agents Chemother. *1*: 433-440.

10. Seligman, S. J. 1966. Methicillin-resistant staphylococci. Genetics of a minority population. J. Gen. Microbiol. *42:* 315-322.
11. Steers, E., E. L. Foltz, and B. S. Graves. 1959. An inocula replicating apparatus for routine testing of bacterial susceptibility to antibiotics. Antibiot. Chemother. *9:* 307-311.
12. Sutter, V. L., and J. A. Washington. 1974. Susceptibility testing of anaerobes. In *Manual of Clinical Microbiology.* 2d ed. E. H. Lennette, E. H. Spaulding, and J. P. Truant (Eds.). American Society for Microbiology, Washington, D. C. pp. 436-438.
13. Tally, F. P., J. G. Bartlett, and S. L. Gorbach. 1975. A practical approach to anaerobic bacteriology for clinical laboratories. In *Technical Improvement Service,* No. 20. American Society of Clinical Pathologists, Chicago, Ill. pp. 42-59.
14. Thornsberry, C., J. Q. Caruthers, and C. N. Baker. 1973. Effect of temperature on the *in vitro* susceptibility of *Staphylococcus aureus* to penicillinase-resistant penicillins. Antimicrob. Agents Chemother. *4:* 263-269.
15. U.S. Department of Health, Education, and Welfare. 1963. *Gonococcus, Procedures for Isolation and Identification.* Public Health Service. Publication No. 499. U.S. Government Printing Office, Washington, D. C. pp. 25-30.
16. Washington, J. A., and A. L. Barry. 1974. Dilution test procedures. In *Manual of Clinical Microbiology.* 2d ed. E. H. Lennette, E. H. Spaulding, and J. P. Truant (Eds.). American Society for Microbiology, Washington, D. C. pp. 410-417.
17. Washington, J. A., W. J. Martin, and P. E. Hermans. 1974. *In vitro* susceptibility of anaerobic bacteria isolated from blood cultures. In *Anaerobic Bacteria: Role in Disease.* A. Balows, R. M. DeHaan, V. R. Dowell, and L. B. Guze (Eds.). Charles C Thomas, Springfield, Ill. pp. 487-496.
18. Washington, J. A., E. Warren, C. T. Dolan, and A. G. Karlson. 1974. Tests to determine the activity of antimicrobial agents. In *Laboratory Procedures in Clinical Microbiology.* J. A. Washington (Ed.). Little, Brown, Boston. pp. 281-340.
19. Wilkins, T. D., and T. Thiel. 1973. Modified broth-disk method for testing the antibiotic susceptibility of anaerobic bacteria. Antimicrob. Agents Chemother. *3:* 350-356.

Chapter **6**

BROTH DILUTION TECHNIQUES

Quantitative susceptibility tests can be performed by diluting the antimicrobic in a nutrient broth rather than in an agar medium as described in the previous chapter. Standard broth dilution techniques are most convenient when only a few strains need to be tested against one or two drugs. With mechanization of the micro-dilution technique, a single isolate can be tested against a fairly large number of drugs with reasonable efficiency. Both types of broth dilution tests permit subculturing after overnight incubation to determine the minimal lethal concentration (MLC) as well as the minimal inhibitory concentration (MIC). When testing microorganisms that require supplementation of the medium with blood or blood products, broth dilution methods are often unsatisfactory because the additives produce a cloudy medium in which microbial growth cannot be detected—a clear broth medium is essential. When the antimicrobics are diluted in an agar medium with such supplements, bacterial growth can be detected on the surface of the agar plates without difficulty.

MACRODILUTION PROCEDURES

Selection of Broth Medium.   Mueller-Hinton broth is preferred for testing the majority of rapid-growing bacterial pathogens since they are able to grow satisfactorily. Other broth media with some-

92

what greater nutritive capacity are recommended only when attempting to test a strain that fails to grow in Mueller-Hinton broth. In that case, a soy bean casein digest (tryptic soy or trypticase soy) broth without dextrose—or a similar medium—may be used. The activity of many antimicrobial agents will be altered significantly by the composition of the broth medium in which the test is performed. Whenever a broth medium other than Mueller-Hinton broth must be used, one or more control strains should be tested against the antimicrobic, which has been diluted in Mueller-Hinton broth as well as in the alternative medium. The differences between the two MICs with the control strains provide information concerning the extent to which this departure from the standard medium might have affected the values obtained with the test strain. The results obtained with the fastidious microorganisms could be adjusted by applying a correction factor based upon the number of dilutions by which the MICs for the control strains are shifted as a result of changing the medium.

Preparation of Antimicrobic Dilutions. Standard broth dilution tests are usually performed in sterile 13-by-100-mm tubes loosely covered with plastic or metal caps or cotton plugs. Each tube receives 1 ml of antimicrobic-containing broth, which, in turn, is diluted further when an equal volume of inoculum is added. If only one microorganism is to be tested, the serial dilutions may be prepared with the standard twofold carry-over dilution technique. Separate pipettes must be employed for each dilution. If several dilution series are to be prepared, the dilution schedule outlined in Table 6-1 is recommended. A single pipette may be used for distributing all diluent and then for adding the stock solution of antimicrobic to the first tube. Thereafter, separate pipettes are used for each block of three dilutions, thus providing an economy of pipettes and minimizing the cumulative error inherent in the standard twofold dilution technique. The antimicrobic dilutions may be prepared in bulk and then 1-ml volumes distributed into the appropriate number of tubes. A control tube containing 1 ml of broth without antimicrobic is always included for each dilution series. A second control tube may be inoculated and held in the refrigerator overnight to serve as a negative control. Appropriate controls should be applied to insure sterility of the broth medium and of the antimicrobic solutions.

Standardization of Inoculum. For each strain to be tested, a standardized inoculum is prepared, following the principles outlined for agar dilution tests (Chapter 5). The inoculum should be diluted to yield a suspension containing approximately 5×10^5

Table 6-1. A Dilution Scheme for Preparation of Broth Dilution Tests

Volume* of Drug Solution and Concentration (μg or IU/ml)	Volume* of Broth Diluent	Concentration (μg or IU/ml) Intermediate	Concentration (μg or IU/ml) Final†	Log$_2$
2 ml 2,000 μg/ml stock	+ 13.62 ml	256 μg/ml	128	7
2 vols 256 μg/ml (above)	+ 2 vols	128 μg/ml	64	6
1 vol 256 μg/ml (above)	+ 3 vols	64 μg/ml	32	5
1 vol 256 μg/ml (above)	+ 7 vols	32 μg/ml	16	4
2 vols 32 μg/ml (above)	+ 2 vols	16 μg/ml	8	3
1 vol 32 μg/ml (above)	+ 3 vols	8 μg/ml	4	2
1 vol 32 μg/ml (above)	+ 7 vols	4 μg/ml	2	1
2 vols 4 μg/ml (above)	+ 2 vols	2 μg/ml	1	0
1 vol 4 μg/ml (above)	+ 3 vols	1 μg/ml	0.5	−1
1 vol 4 μg/ml (above)	+ 7 vols	0.5 μg/ml	0.25	−2
2 vols 0.5 μg/ml (above)	+ 2 vols	0.25 μg/ml	0.125	−3
1 vol 0.5 μg/ml (above)	+ 3 vols	0.125 μg/ml	0.063	−4
1 vol 0.5 μg/ml (above)	+ 7 vols	0.063 μg/ml	0.031	−5
etc.		etc.	etc.	etc.

* Any multiple of the volumes in the table may be used according to the number of tests being made, i.e., 0.5 ml vol suffices for 2 tests, 1 vol for 4 tests, 4 ml vol for 8 tests, etc.

† The final concentration is obtained after 1 ml of the intermediate dilution is further diluted with an equal volume of inoculum.

CFU/ml rather than 5×10^6 CFU/ml, as recommended for the agar dilution technique. A satisfactory inoculum is generally obtained by preparing a 1:2,000 dilution of a stationary-phase broth culture (overnight, 4-5-ml broth cultures or four-to-six-hour, 0.5-ml broth cultures of enteric bacilli, *Pseudomonas aeruginosa*, and *Staphylococcus aureus*) or by preparing a 1:200 dilution of a suspension after adjusting to match the turbidity of a MacFarland 0.5 standard. The inoculum is diluted in the same broth medium used for the test (generally Mueller-Hinton broth) but the initial growth can be obtained in a more nutritive medium, such as trypticase soy broth or brain-heart infusion broth.

Inoculation and Incubation. The tubes containing 1-ml volumes of the serially diluted antimicrobic and the appropriate control tubes are each inoculated with an equal volume of the standardized cell suspension. This should be completed within 20 minutes after the inoculum is standardized since the microorganisms might begin to multiply if the broth suspension is held any longer. The tubes are then gently mixed and allowed to incubate 16 to 18 hours at 35°C. Incubation in an atmosphere of increased CO_2 is not recommended unless essential for growth of the microorganism being tested, and then appropriate controls must be instituted (as with agar dilution tests).

Reading Test Results. The lowest concentration of antimicrobic producing complete inhibition of growth represents the MIC. A very faint haziness or small clump of questionable growth is generally disregarded, whereas a large cluster of growth or definite turbidity is considered evidence that the drug has failed to inhibit growth completely at that concentration. The appearance of the positive and negative control tubes should always be considered before selecting the end-point. The minimal concentration required for a lethal effect (MLC) may be determined by transferring a measured volume of broth for each tube showing inhibited growth to an antimicrobic-free medium (see page 100).

MICRODILUTION PROCEDURES

The broth dilution technique described above can be adapted to the microtitration techniques that were originally developed for serologic procedures. Trays or plates containing eight rows of small, flat-bottomed or V-shaped cups can be used as if they were racks of small (0.1-ml) test tubes. To each well, 50-μl (0.05-ml) volumes of broth are added, using one of the several varieties of dropping pipettes currently available. Special calibrated loops may then be used to transfer 50 μl of the antimicrobic stock solution to the first well in each row and then mixed by twirling the loops. After the mixing, 50 μl is transferred from the first well to the second well, and this process is continued in order to prepare serial dilutions of the antimicrobic. By holding several loops in the same hand or by using a special handle, as many as 12 diluters may be manipulated at the same time. In this way as many as 12 different antimicrobics can be diluted serially at the same time. Several mechanized systems have been devised to permit preparation of the antimicrobic dilution in a semi-automated fashion. Those semi-automated systems that have been evaluated properly appear to be capable of producing accurate and precise dilutions. However, as with all complex mechanical devices, malfunctions do occur—and often enough to necessitate continual monitoring of samples from each batch of trays in order to control the test system properly.

Storage of Microdilution Trays. Microdilutions of antimicrobics may be prepared each day so as to provide enough trays for the number of strains to be tested that day. With semi-automated equipment for preparing microdilutions, it is possible to prepare large numbers of trays at one time and not practical to provide freshly diluted trays each day. Consequently, a system is called for by which the trays may be stored for short periods of time. The following procedure has been found satisfactory.

The trays are stacked as they are prepared, with an empty tray on top. Each tray fits on top of another snugly enough to provide a cover that helps to minimize evaporation and airborne contamination. A stack of from five to ten trays is placed in a plastic bag that is then sealed so as to provide an airtight container. The bag of trays may then be frozen at –20°C or lower. A regular household freezer is satisfactory, but freezers with automatic defrost should be avoided since there may be enough fluctuation in the temperature to hasten deterioration of some of the more labile antimicrobics. An ultracold freezer (–60°C or under) may also be used for short-term storage of the microdilution trays. When handled in this way, the microdilution trays may be stored for two to three weeks, ready for use when needed. Once a stack of trays is removed from the freezer, they should be allowed to warm to room temperature before the bag is opened. Unused thawed trays should be discarded, never refrozen.

Antimicrobic stock solutions are often prepared in bulk, and aliquots are frozen until needed. If such frozen stock solutions are used for preparing microdilution trays that are refrozen for short-term storage, the drug will be subjected to two freeze-thaw cycles, a procedure that is often discouraged on the grounds that it may hasten inactivation of the labile drugs. However, limited experience to date suggests that two freeze-thaw cycles might not be too detrimental to most antimicrobics. Thus, the use of stored stock solutions may be suggested if adequate controls are applied to detect inactivation of the stored antimicrobic dilutions.

Microdilution trays containing appropriate concentrations of antimicrobial agents may be purchased through Micro-Media Systems, Inc. (Palo Alto, Calif.), which has established regional production centers throughout the United States and Canada. Each center is capable of providing a continually replenished supply of frozen microdilution trays that are simply held in the freezer of the clinical laboratory, ready for inoculation when needed.

Inoculation of Microdilution Trays. The inoculum is standardized in the same way as described for the macro- broth dilution technique. Each well then receives 50 μl of the adjusted inoculum, resulting in a twofold reduction of the final concentration of antimicrobic in each well. Reliable results have been reported when the inoculum is distributed by use of a disposable 50-μl dropping pipette (Cooke Engineering, Alexandria, Va.).[15,16] A multiple-inoculum replicator has been developed. It consists of a metal plate containing wire prongs that will inoculate all the wells on one tray simultaneously. Since each wire prong is said to deliver about 1 μl, the inoculum must be standardized to give a density 50 times greater than that required when 50-μl drops are added to each well. Although an early model of this wire-pronged inoculator has been found to be unsatisfactory,[15,16] similar devices have been used with apparent success by other investigators. Micro-Media Systems, Inc., provides its customers with an attractive inoculator that is said to deliver about 5 μl to each well. Regardless of what type inoculator is used, each individual device should be carefully evaluated before being accepted for routine use, and its precision and accuracy must be monitored regularly. When an inoculator is to be used, the final volume of antimicrobic in the microdilution trays should be 100 μl, rather than the 50 μl prescribed when a dropping pipette is used.

Incubation of Trays. After being inoculated, the microdilution trays are covered with sealing tape in order to minimize evaporation. The trays are then allowed to incubate at 35°C. They must be stacked no more than two high on each shelf, because a center tray would reach incubator temperature much more slowly than those on the top and bottom. Furthermore, the wells on the sides would come to temperature faster than those in the center. This delay in equilibration of temperature might very well influence the final result with some drugs. For general routine susceptibility testing, trays are often stacked four or five deep, and in incubators with proper humidity control the sealing tape is often omitted.[15]

Reading Test Results. After from 16 to 18 hours of incubation, the microdilution trays may be examined on a viewer after the sealing tape has been removed. The end-point is taken as the lowest concentration at which the microorganisms do not produce visible turbidity or clusters of growth. The microorganism is considered resistant to the concentration in which there is a definite turbidity, a single cluster of growth 2 mm or greater in diameter, or more than one cluster of growth (even if it is less than 2 mm in diameter).

Modification for Testing Anaerobes. Anaerobic microorganisms may be tested with the microdilution technique.[12,13] However, it is difficult to evaluate the accuracy and precision of such an approach, because of the limited number of adequate studies reported in the current literature. The inoculum is prepared and antimicrobics diluted in an appropriate broth medium (such as Brucella broth, Schaedler's broth, or brain-heart infusion broth) supplemented with menadione (5 μg/ml) and hemin (0.1 μg/ml). Sufficient comparative studies have not yet been carried out to support the selection of a single standard medium; each medium has its own advantages and disadvantages, and the final decision depends on the individual investigator's previous experiences with the types of anaerobes being studied. The antimicrobic dilutions may be prepared in advance and stored frozen. At least two hours before use, the trays should be removed from the freezer and placed directly into an anaerobic glove box (5% CO_2, 10% H_2, and 85% N_2). This procedure reduces the amount of oxygen that has penetrated the medium and the plastic trays. The remaining steps are carried out as described above for testing the aerobes, except that the entire process is performed inside an anaerobic glove box. Most anaerobes can be tested in anaerobic jars, e.g., Gas-Pak jars.

Modification for Testing Hemophilus influenzae. The microdilution technique may be used for studying the susceptibility of *H. influenzae* to a variety of antimicrobics. Tests against ampicillin are of particular interest.[14] The Mueller-Hinton broth may be supplemented with 5% (v/v) peptic digest of blood, as described for the agar dilution procedure. In practice, the antimicrobic may be diluted in Mueller-Hinton broth with 10% (v/v) peptic digest of blood that is later diluted 1:2 when the trays are inoculated. The inoculum is prepared by suspending the growth from an overnight chocolate agar plate directly into Mueller-Hinton broth. This suspension is adjusted to match the turbidity of a MacFarland 0.5 turbidity standard (about 10^8 CFU/ml) and is further diluted 10^{-4} in Mueller-Hinton broth so as to obtain a suspension containing 10^4 CFU/ml. The density of inoculum actually obtained with randomly sampled test strains should be monitored regularly, as described for agar dilution tests. Each well is inoculated with 0.05 ml of this suspension delivered from a dropping pipette. After 24 hours at 35°C, the end-points are determined by examination with reflected light. Ampicillin-resistant strains of *H. influenzae* frequently demonstrate "soft" end-points, in which the amount of growth decreases gradually over two or three dilution steps, whereas susceptible strains tend to give more clear-cut results.

The density of the inoculum and the time of incubation have profound effects on the final end-point obtained with ampicillin.[14] However, with the above-mentioned procedure, ampicillin-resistant and ampicillin-susceptible strains are readily separated; the latter being inhibited by less than 1 μg/ml and the former generally requiring at least 8 μg/ml for inhibition.

BACTERICIDAL ACTIVITY OF ANTIMICROBICS

The broth dilution techniques described above determine the minimal inhibitory concentration (MIC). At concentrations near the MIC end-point, inhibition of growth is usually reversible and viable microorganisms can be recovered when the concentration of drug is reduced to sub-inhibitory levels (as by dilution). With many antimicrobics, an irreversible inhibition (a "killing" effect) may be observed at concentrations slightly greater than that required for inhibition. In a limited number of clinical situations, chemotherapy should be adjusted to obtain a concentration at the site of infection that exceeds that required for a lethal effect *in vitro*. This is especially important when the host's defense mechanisms are severely compromised in such a way that the microorganisms might not be cleared from the site of infection although their multiplication is inhibited by the chemotherapeutic agent. In such situations it would be appropriate to determine *in vitro* the minimal lethal concentration (MLC) as well as the MIC. Unfortunately, there are no uniformly accepted techniques for determining the lethal effect, and there are unresolved differences of opinion among investigators accustomed to using different methods for doing the same type of test. The following paragraphs outline two generally accepted methods by which a bactericidal activity can be measured *in vitro*.[1]

The MLC may be defined arbitrarily as the lowest *concentration* of drug that produces a minimum number or defined proportion of viable survivors after incubation for a fixed time under a given set of conditions. Alternatively, the lethal activity may be expressed as the *rate* of killing by a fixed concentration of antimicrobic measured by determining the number of survivors at various time intervals after inoculation. Some controversy centers around the exact details by which one defines the arbitrarily selected parameters of such tests, but the basic principles outlined in the following sections are generally accepted by most investigators.

Determination of MLCs. By incorporating the following few additional procedures, the standard broth dilution techniques described above may be used to determine the MLC as well as the MIC:

1. At the time of inoculation a viable cell count should be performed. This can be done easily by preparing a 1:100 and 1:1,000 dilution of the control tube after inoculation and then spreading 0.1 ml of each dilution over the surface of separate blood agar plates. After overnight incubation, the colonies are counted and the inoculum is calculated from the plate showing from 50 to 200 colonies.
2. After 16 to 18 hours of incubation, the MIC is determined as described previously. Each tube or well showing no visible evidence of microbial growth is then subcultured to a quadrant of blood agar plate to determine whether viable organisms are present. Some investigators prefer to subculture 0.1-ml aliquots to obtain a degree of reliability in counting the number of survivors present near the end-point. Others prefer to transfer 0.01-ml volumes by the use of a calibrated loop, with inevitable loss of accuracy but significant gain in efficiency. Carry-over of antimicrobic onto the agar plate is reduced by subculturing the smaller volume. In general, satisfactory results are obtained if approximately 5% to 10% of the total volume in each tube or microdilution well is spread over one-half or one-fourth of a blood agar plate. Antimicrobic carry-over in such large volumes is reduced in concentration by diffusion into the adjacent agar medium. Because of this diffusion, the number of samples spread over sections of one blood agar plate must be held to a minimum.
3. After 18 to 24 hours of incubation, the subcultures are examined and the number of colony-forming units determined. The MLC may be defined as the lowest concentration that results in a 99.9% kill. That is, no more than 0.1% of the viable cells in the primary inoculum are able to survive and grow under the test conditions. Thus if each tube was shown to have received 10^5 CFU/ml, a lethal effect would be attributed to those concentrations of antimicrobic that contain no more than 100 survivors per ml, that is, ten colonies or fewer from 0.1-ml aliquots or one colony or fewer from 0.01-ml samples. Because of the anticipated sampling error, the latter example is not likely to yield statistically reliable results, whereas the transfer of larger volumes is more likely to give reproducible results when the number of survivors is relatively small.

Killing Rate. In some experimental situations, the lethal activity may be expressed best in terms of the *rate* of killing by fixed concentrations of antimicrobic. Such an approach is particularly useful for comparing the activity of two or more antimicrobics or combination of antimicrobics. For each drug or combination of drugs, a tube is prepared with 10 ml of broth containing the antimicrobic(s) at a predetermined concentration (generally approaching the average blood level expected during therapy with the usual dosage or just above the expected inhibitory concentration). For testing most enteric bacilli or staphylococci, Mueller-Hinton broth is an appropriate medium. All antimicrobic-containing media and a control tube with 10 ml of broth without antimicrobic are inoculated so as to give a final inoculum of about 10^5 microorganisms per ml in each tube. The growth dynamics are then studied during incubation at 35°C.

Immediately after inoculation, and periodically thereafter, each tube is mixed and samples are withdrawn. Suitable dilutions of each sample are prepared and colony counts performed. The total number of survivors should be determined at least after 0, 4, and 24 hours of incubation. More frequent counts are required occasionally, and in some cases 48-hour or even 72-hour determinations may be indicated. The actual colony counts may be performed in a number of ways, but generally it is possible to prepare rather broad dilution steps followed by surface plating onto any nutritionally adequate agar medium. Multiple replicates are not essential since logarithmic decreases in the number of viable cells are being sought.

The results are presented graphically by plotting the total number of viable cells on a logarithmic scale against the hours of incubation, as displayed in Figure 6-1. By comparing the rate of decline in the number of survivors observed with the different drugs or combination of drugs, it is possible to identify the most rapidly lethal antimicrobic under these test conditions. An early decrease in the number of survivors may be followed by a marked increase in the number of viable cells. This might be due to the selection of resistant variants or to the partial inactivation of the antimicrobial agent during incubation, or to both factors.

Some antimicrobics are reversibly bound to serum proteins, thus decreasing the concentration of antimicrobic free to act on the microorganisms. With such drugs the MIC is increased if *in vitro* tests are carried out with added blood or blood products. Since the protein binding is a reversible phenomenon, the antimicrobic in the pool of unbound drug is replenished as it is removed by combining with the microorganism. Although it is difficult to determine the clinical significance of protein-binding experiments that are carried out *in vitro* under rather static conditions, it is clear that certain antimicrobics are markedly affected by the presence of serum proteins added to an *in vitro* test system. Some investigators prefer to

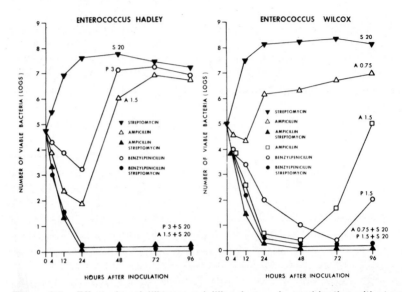

Figure 6-1. Effect of penicillin or ampicillin, alone or in combination with streptomycin, on the number of viable enterococci of two strains, during incubation at 37°C for four days. (From M. Sonne and E. Jawetz. 1968. Appl. Microbiol. *16:* 647.)

test all antimicrobics in normal human serum or in broth with 50% serum added because it presumably mimics the *in vivo* situations more closely. Since serum itself is a variable product, samples from a large number of healthy individuals should be pooled. It is known that different batches of normal serum may have some bactericidal activity against some strains of bacteria.[16] This bactericidal activity is complement dependent and declines during storage. In practice, pooled samples of human serum are stored for various periods of time before being used, and appropriate controls must be incorporated when the addition of human serum to any *in vitro* test system is considered necessary. If a sample of pooled serum has been found to inhibit the microorganism being tested, it may be heat inactivated at 56°C for 30 minutes to eliminate the complement-dependent bactericidal activity, which may be difficult to distinguish from the bactericidal activity of the antimicrobic being tested.

SERUM BACTERICIDAL TESTS

The standard broth dilution procedure described in this chapter may be modified in order to determine directly the bactericidal activity of serum from patients being treated with one or more antimicrobics. Dilutions of the serum are tested against the patient's own infecting microorganism. Serum bactericidal tests are helpful in obtaining an appropriate dosage schedule. The methods for determining serum bactericidal activity have been modified many times since the procedure was first described in 1947 by Schlichter et al.[7,9,10] The following is one method for performing the serum bactericidal test. It may be adapted for use in a microdilution procedure.

In principle, the standard broth dilution technique for determining the MLC is adapted, using the patient's serum sample rather than the antimicrobics, and the results are expressed as the highest dilution of serum that demonstrates a lethal effect. If the dilutions were prepared in broth, each tube would provide decreasing amounts of human serum, which would tend to complicate the interpretation of tests with those drugs that are highly protein bound. To hold that one variable constant, the patient's serum is diluted with inactivated normal human pooled serum so that every tube contains the same amount of serum protein. To conserve diluent, the test is carried out in one-half the volume recommended for the standard broth dilution test.

1. A recent bacterial isolate from the patient is transferred and stored at –20°C or lower in a suitably stabilized broth medium, such as trypticase soy broth with 15% (v/v) glycerol. Just before the test is to be run, the stored culture is transferred to an appropriately nutrient agar medium, and after overnight incubation four or five isolated colonies are transferred to Mueller-Hinton broth (other broth media may be used if required for rapid growth of the test strain). The broth subculture then serves as inoculum after five or six hours of incubation and appropriate dilution.

2. Serum samples are collected from the patient before therapy has begun and again 24 hours after treatment has been initiated. If intermittent therapy is being given, two samples should be collected to estimate the lowest and highest levels; one sample is collected just before a dose is given (lowest level) and the other about one hour after intramuscular injection or immediately after intravenous infusion (peak level). Once separated from the clot, serum samples may be stored at –20°C for several days without loss of antimicrobic activity.

3. For each serum sample, twofold dilutions are prepared in 0.5-ml volumes with inactivated normal human pooled serum as diluent, the first tube containing 0.5 ml of the patient's serum (to be diluted 1:2 when inoculated).

4. The patient's isolate is then diluted in Mueller-Hinton broth or other appropriate broth so as to obtain about 2×10^5 CFU/ml. Viable cell counts are made at that time, to establish the initial inoculum density. Each tube is inoculated with 0.5 ml of this standardization cell suspension. Three controls are also inoculated:

   (1) 0.5 ml of the pooled serum diluent,
   (2) 0.5 ml of broth with no serum, and
   (3) if available, 0.5 ml of pretreatment serum. The latter is required to exclude inhibition by normal bactericidal mechanisms, but in practice it is often impossible to obtain such a serum sample before some chemotherapy has been initiated.

5. Because of the turbidity inherent in certain serum samples, inhibitory levels are often impossible to determine and thus the bactericidal activity is routinely determined, as described earlier in this chapter.

6. After appropriate incubation of the subcultures, the maximal dilution of serum that gives a 99.9% kill is determined for each serum sample. Interpretation may have

to be individualized according to the nature and severity of the illness and the toxicity of the drug. In general, dosage is considered to be adequate if a bactericidal activity can be demonstrated at a dilution of 1:8 or 1:16.[6]

REFERENCES

1. Barry, A. L., and L. D. Sabath. 1974. Special tests: Bactericidal activity and activity of antimicrobics in combination. In *Manual of Clinical Microbiology*, 2d ed. E. H. Lennette, E. H. Spaulding, and J. P. Truant (Eds.). American Society for Microbiology, Washington, D. C. pp. 431-435.
2. Gavan, T. L., and M. A. Town. 1970. A microdilution method for antibiotic susceptibility testing: An evaluation. Am. J. Clin. Pathol. 53: 880-885.
3. Gavan, T. L., and D. A. Butler. 1974. An automated microdilution method for antimicrobial testing. In *Current Techniques for Antibiotic Susceptibility Testing*. A. Balows (Ed.). Charles C Thomas, Springfield, Ill. pp. 88-93.
4. Gerlach, E. H. 1974. Microdilution: A comparative study. In *Current Techniques for Antibiotic Susceptibility Testing*. A. Balows (Ed.). Charles C Thomas, Springfield, Ill. pp. 63-76.
5. Gerlach, E. H., R. J. Taylor, and B. Bauman. 1969. The comparison of a manual and an automated method of routinely performed serial dilution antibiotic sensitivity tests in a large hospital. Am. J. Clin. Pathol. 52: 748-750.
6. Klostersky, J., D. Daneau, G. Swings, and D. Weerts. 1974. Antibacterial activity in serum and urine as a therapeutic guide in bacterial infections. J. Infect. Dis. 129: 187-193.
7. Pien, F. D., and K. L. Vosti. 1974. Variation in performance of the serum bactericidal test. Antimicrob. Agents Chemother. 6: 330-333.
8. Pien, F. D., R. D. Williams, and K. L. Vosti. 1975. Comparison of broth and human serum as the diluent in the serum bactericidal test. Antimicrob. Agents Chemother. 7: 113-114.
9. Schlichter, J. G., and H. MacLean. 1947. A method of determining the effective therapeutic level in the treatment of subacute bacterial endocarditis with penicillin. Am. Heart J. 34: 209-211.
10. Schlichter, J. G., H. MacLean, and A. Malzer. 1949. Effective penicillin therapy in subacute bacterial endocarditis and other chronic infections. Am. J. Med. Sci. 217: 600-608.
11. Sonne, M., and E. Jawetz. 1968. Comparison of ampicillin and benzyl penicillin on enterococci *in vitro*. Appl. Microbiol. 16: 645-648.
12. Stalons, D. R., and C. Thornsberry, 1975. Broth-dilution method for determining the antibiotic susceptibility of anaerobic bacteria. Antimicrob. Agents Chemother. 7: 15-21.
13. Thornsberry, C. 1975. Antimicrobial susceptibility testing of anaerobes. In *Technical Improvement Service*, vol. 20. American Society of Clinical Pathologists, Chicago, Ill., pp. 60-68.
14. Thornsberry, C., and L. A. Kirven. 1974. Antimicrobial susceptibility of *Haemophilus influenzae*. Antimicrob. Agents Chemother. 6: 620-624.
15. Tilton, R. C., L. Lieberman, and E. H. Gerlach. 1973. Microdilution antibiotic susceptibility test: Examination of certain variables. Appl. Microbiol. 26: 658-665.
16. Tilton, R. C., and L. Newberg. 1974. Standardization of microdilution susceptibility test. In *Current Techniques for Antibiotic Susceptibility Testing*. A. Balows (Ed.). Charles C Thomas, Springfield, Ill. pp. 77-87.
17. Traub, W. H. 1969. Assay of the antibiotic activity of serum. Appl. Microbiol. 18: 51-56.

Chapter 7

METHODS FOR TESTING
ANTIMICROBIC COMBINATIONS

The clinical advantages of chemotherapy with combinations of two or more antimicrobial agents are not well documented, except in the treatment of tuberculosis and enterococcal endocarditis. Combinations are often used in the treatment of other serious infections in an attempt to exploit the phenomenon of synergism, especially to obtain a rapid bactericidal effect. In tuberculosis, two or three drugs are given together to prevent the selection of resistant variants that occur rapidly during single drug therapy. Enterococcal endocarditis is often treated with benzylpenicillin or ampicillin in very high doses or in combination with one of the aminocyclitols (streptomycin, kanamycin, or gentamicin). The latter combination often provides a markedly increased bactericidal activity against most strains of enterococci.

A combination is considered to be synergistic when the effect observed with a combination is greater than the sum of the effects observed with the two drugs independently. Many other combinations of antimicrobial agents are only additive or indifferent, that is, the combined effect is equal to the sum of the effects observed with the two drugs tested separately or equal to that of the most active drug in the combination. Some drug combinations are clearly antagonistic, that is, the combination is less effective than the most active drug in the combination. One of the important reasons for determining the *in vitro* effect of antimicrobic combinations is to avoid antagonism.

Although synergistically active antimicrobics may display a slightly reduced inhibitory concentration when tested in combination, the lethal activity of the combination is often enhanced to a much greater extent. For that reason, methods for testing combination of antimicrobics should determine the lethal activity as well as the inhibitory effect.

AGAR DIFFUSION TECHNIQUES

Bacteriostatic Effect. Two drugs in combination can be studied qualitatively by a simple agar diffusion technique.[4,6] Filter paper (Schleicher and Schuell No. 740E) is cut into strips approximately 4 cm by 0.9 cm, sterilized by autoclaving, and dried. Each of two filter paper strips is then dipped into different antimicrobic solutions, drained, and applied directly to an inoculated agar plate. The strips are placed at a 90° angle, with ends just touching. After overnight incubation, the plates are examined for a zone of inhibition around each strip (Fig. 7-1). At the point where these two zones

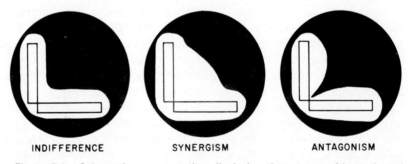

INDIFFERENCE   SYNERGISM   ANTAGONISM

Figure 7-1. Schematic representation displaying three types of bacteriostatic results with combinations of antimicrobial agents tested by the agar diffusion technique.

meet, the two drugs are present in decreasing concentrations. If the two drugs are indifferent, the two zones will meet to form a right angle, or, at most, the angle may be slightly rounded. Synergism is shown by an inhibition of growth within the angle where both drugs are present in sub-inhibitory concentrations. Antagonism is shown when the zone of growth is indented inside the zone where inhibition should occur.

This approach may be useful for screening drug combinations that display marked synergy or antagonism; the test is neither quantitative nor is it particularly sensitive to the subtle effects sometimes seen with drug combinations. The success or failure of the paper-strip method is dependent upon achieving the proper concentration of antimicrobic in each strip, which is best determined for each drug combination by trial and error for a given test organism.

Bactericidal Effect. Drug combinations can be tested qualitatively by the cellophane transfer technique of Chabbert et al.[3,6,16] Glass cylinders with flat ground rims about 6 cm deep and of a diameter sufficient to fit inside a petri plate are required. A tambourine is prepared by attaching a cellophane disc to the flat ground ends of the cylinder. The cellophane should be tested for permeability to nutrients so that when it is laid onto a nutrient agar plate and seeded with a bacterial culture, growth should be the same as that observed when the agar plate is inoculated directly. Since cellophane stretches when moistened, it must be kept moist at all times. If allowed to dry, it will wrinkle and prove unsatisfactory for transfer of bacterial cultures. A cellophane disc is boiled in distilled water for about ten minutes and then stretched over one end of the glass cylinder and fixed into position with two rubber bands. The excess cellophane is trimmed and the tambourine checked to be sure the cellophane is flat and taut. The tambourine is placed onto a disc of moist blotting paper in a suitable container for autoclaving. Thus prepared, the tambourine may be stored as long as the cellophane inside the container remains moist and smooth.

To perform the test, filter-paper strips (Schleicher and Schuell No. 740E) are dipped into the appropriate antimicrobic solutions, drained, and applied at right angles to the surface of an uninoculated agar plate (Fig. 7-2). The drugs are then allowed to diffuse overnight at 35°C. After the location and identification of each strip is marked, the strips are removed and discarded. A sterile tambourine is then applied to the medium—without trapping any air bubbles between the medium and the cellophane—and excess moisture is removed by drying at 35°C, about 30 minutes. The cellophane is flooded with 1 ml of an overnight broth culture diluted 1:10 or 1:100, and excess fluid is removed by aspiration, followed by another 30-minute drying period. The plate is then inverted and allowed to incubate with the medium resting on the glass cylinder standing on clean blotting paper on the incubator shelf without a lid. Drying after inoculation and incubation of the

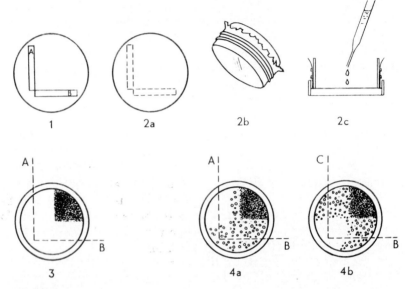

1. Prediffusion.
2. (a) Prediffused plate, (b) tambour, (c) tambour applied receiving inoculum.
3. Primary growth.
4. Secondary growth after transfer to antibiotic-free medium. (a) Antibiotics A and B combined = antagonism; (b) antibiotics C and B combined = synergism.
   NOTE: A is a bactericidal antibiotic for this organism; B and C are bacteriostatic alone but kill the organism when combined.

Figure 7-2. Diagrammatic outline of cellophane transfer technique for detecting the bactericidal effect of antimicrobial agents in combination. (From E. J. Stokes. 1975. *Clinical Bacteriology*. 4th ed. Williams & Wilkins, Baltimore. p. 244.)

inverted plate without a lid is important to prevent excess moisture from spreading over the cellophane surface.

As soon as primary growth becomes visible (6 to 18 hours), the tambourine is transferred to a fresh, well-dried blood agar plate and re-incubated as before. The second plate is examined after overnight incubation for secondary growth inside the zone of inhibition, representing viable cells that were inhibited but not killed. In this way, it is possible to detect a bactericidal synergism or antagonism between the two drugs much the same as described above.

Lorian and Fodor[12] have described a modification of the cellophane transfer technique in which the cellophane tambourine is replaced by a membrane filter and tetrazolium chloride (TTC) is incorporated into the Mueller-Hinton agar base. When growth of the microorganisms has occurred, the TTC is reduced to a red formazan, which sharply contrasts with the white membrane where a bactericidal effect has occurred.

BROTH DILUTION TECHNIQUES

Although agar diffusion methods are reasonably simple to perform, they do not provide the quantitative information that can be derived from broth dilution techniques. Either one of the two methods for measuring the bactericidal activity of antimicrobics can be adapted for testing combinations of drugs.

Test Procedure. For studying drug combinations, the broth dilution technique described in the previous chapter may be modified in the following way. Both drugs are serially diluted in large volumes and then combined in a checkerboard fashion so as to obtain many possible combinations of drug concentrations and one series of doubling dilutions for each antimicrobic alone (Table 7-1). The tubes are then all inoculated with a standardized suspension of the test organism, and the number of viable cells in each tube is determined by performing colony counts on the diluted inoculum. After from 16 to 18 hours, inhibitory end-points are read for each drug alone and for each drug in the presence of the other drug. Subcultures of tubes or wells showing inhibited growth are made to determine the MLCs (as described in Chapter 6) if lethal end-points are desired.

Table 7-1. Sample Arrangement of Test Tubes for Testing an Enterococcus against Combinations of Gentamicin and Benzylpenicillin

Final Concentration (μg/ml) of:
Gentamicin/Benzylpenicillin

0/ 0	0.5/ 0	1.0/ 0	2.0/ 0	4.0/ 0
0/ 0.25	0.5/ 0.25	1.0/ 0.25	2.0/ 0.25	4.0/ 0.25
0/ 0.5	0.5/ 0.5	1.0/ 0.5	2.0/ 0.5	4.0/ 0.5
0/ 1.0	0.5/ 1.0	1.0/ 1.0	2.0/ 1.0	4.0/ 1.0
0/ 2.0	0.5/ 2.0	1.0/ 2.0	2.0/ 2.0	4.0/ 2.0
0/ 4.0	0.5/ 4.0	1.0/ 4.0	2.0/ 4.0	4.0/ 4.0
0/ 8.0	0.5/ 8.0	1.0/ 8.0	2.0/ 8.0	4.0/ 8.0
0/16	0.5/16	1.0/16	2.0/16	4.0/16
0/32	0.5/32	1.0/32	2.0/32	4.0/32
0/64	0.5/64	1.0/64	2.0/64	4.0/64

* 0.25 ml of a solution containing 4 times the desired final concentration is added to each tube in a row (0 = broth without drug). All 50 tubes are then inoculated each with 0.5 ml of appropriately diluted cultures, resulting in a 1:4 dilution of the drugs.

Analysis of Results. To determine whether there is evidence of synergistic inhibition or killing, the results are displayed graphically as shown in Figure 7-3, an isobologram. To construct an

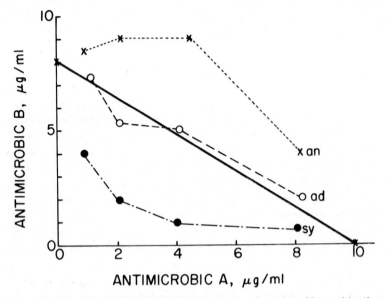

Figure 7-3. Isobolograms displaying three types of results with combinations of antimicrobics. When the minimal inhibitory concentrations of a combination of two antimicrobics fall along a line demarcated by the minimal inhibitory concentration of each agent by itself (8 μg/ml for B and 10 μg/ml for A), the effect is additive (*curve ad*). Bowing toward the origin indicates synergism (curve sy), whereas bowing outward, away from the origin, is consistent with antagonism (curve an). (From P. D. Hoeprich, (Ed.). 1972. *Infectious Diseases*, 1st ed. Harper & Row Inc., Hagerstown, Md., p. 203.)

isobologram, the MIC or MLC for one drug is plotted on the horizontal scale and the same end-point for the other drug alone is plotted on the vertical scale, using arithmetic scales intersecting at a zero value. For each concentration of antimicrobic plotted on the horizontal scale, an MIC of the vertical antimicrobic is determined and plotted on the isobologram. To check the proper location of points, plot each concentration of antimicrobic on the vertical scale, and the MIC or MLC for the drug on the horizontal scale. In this way a series of points is determined and can be joined by a curved line originating at the MIC or MLC for one drug and terminating for the value determined for the other drug alone. A straight line joining the values obtained with each drug separately represents an isobol that indicates an additive effect between the two antimicrobics. Antagonism is indicated by an isobol that bows upward away from the coordinant; a bowing toward the coordinant indicates synergism. Technical problems could easily produce an isobol that deviates from the straight line by a single dilution step, and thus a deviation of two or more dilution steps is often required before a combination of drugs is labeled synergistic or antagonistic.

The actual construction of the isobologram can be simplified by calculating the fractional inhibitory concentration (FIC) or fractional lethal concentration (FLC) of each antimicrobic. The FIC is calculated by dividing the concentration of antimicrobic present in the combination by the amount of that drug that would be required for inhibition by itself. In this way, the activity of each drug alone is given a value of 1, and the fraction of that drug required to inhibit growth in the presence of increasing concentrations of the second drug is expressed as a fraction. The reverse combinations are also calculated using the MIC or MLC for the second drug alone as the denominator. This permits construction of isobolograms with simplified arithmetic scales ranging from 0 to 1. When the effect of the two compounds is additive, the points fall on a straight line, connecting unity on the ordinate with unity on the abscissa. Deviation to the left of this theoretical line indicates synergism, and deviations to the right represent interference or antagonism between the antimicrobics. By drawing intersecting straight lines through the experimental points, one arrives at a point where the combined fractional inhibitory concentrations reach a maximal synergism or antagonism. At that point, the FIC for one drug added to the FIC for the other drug can be used as a single figure that denotes the degree of synergism or antagonism by a combination of antimicrobics. The sum of FIC values at the point of maximal effectiveness should approach unity when the inhibitors are additive—the smaller the number the greater the degree of synergism. In addition to ease of plotting, calculations based on fractional inhibitory concentrations are advantageous since they minimize to a considerable extent the effects of biological variability. That is to say, the absolute levels required for inhibition of a microorganism may differ from day to day, but the FIC calculated from data obtained in one experiment should be more nearly replicable.

The construction of an isobologram requires a large number of test tubes and a considerable amount of time. Adaptation to a microdilution technique with mechanization makes it much more practical for large studies or for testing isolates from individual patients.

COMPARISON OF KILLING RATES

Another approach to the problem of testing drug combinations is to document the rates of killing by concentrations of the two drugs singly and in combination, as described in the previous section of this chapter. The results may be presented graphically, as demonstrated in Figure 7-4. The concentration of each drug is fixed,

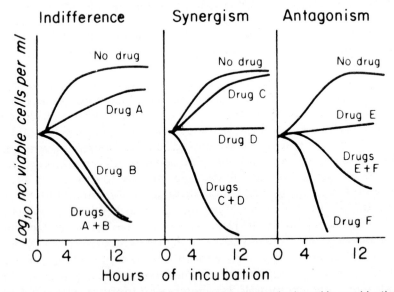

Figure 7-4. Rate of killing with antimicrobial agents singly and in combination. Schematic representation showing three different types of results. (From A. L. Barry and L. D. Sabath. 1974. *Manual of Clinical Microbiology.* 2d Ed. E. H. Lennette, E. H. Spaulding, and J. P. Truant (Eds.). American Society for Microbiology, Washington, D. C. p. 434.)

usually at a level that corresponds to the average blood level or at a concentration near the expected inhibitory concentration. If the rate of decline in number of survivors in the presence of both drugs is nearly the same as that observed with the more active drug of the combination alone, the combination is said to be indifferent. If the two drugs in combination are significantly less active than either one of the drugs alone, the combination is said to be antagonistic. Synergism is displayed when the rate of killing is much more rapid with both drugs in combination than with either drug alone. In all cases a control with no drug is essential for interpreting the test results.

The labor involved in multiple-colony counts makes this approach prohibitive for routine use in most clinical laboratories. Bulger and Nielson[2] have shown that the establishment of killing curves may be simplified considerably. They recommended that 10-ml volumes of Mueller-Hinton broth containing the antimicrobics to be studied alone and in combinations should be inoculated with approximately 5×10^5 microorganisms per ml. After removal of a sample for an initial estimate of viable cells, the test tubes are incubated at 35°C for four hours, at which time a second colony count is performed. A platinum loop calibrated to deliver 0.001 ml is used to perform the colony counts. Care must be taken to insert the loop vertically into the test culture just below the surface, avoiding transfer on the wire above the loop. This loopful of broth is then seeded into a melted and cooled agar medium, which is mixed and poured into a standard petri plate. After appropriate incubation, the colony counts are removed from the incubator and the total number of colony-forming units (CFU) determined. An electronic colony counter and recording device allows rapid and reasonably accurate counting of as many as 600 colonies per petri plate, provided that the colonies are evenly distributed throughout the agar. If there is no growth, one can be certain only that there are fewer than 1,000 surviving CFU/ml. With an initial inoculum of 500,000 CFU/ml this is usually sufficient to determine significant synergism or antagonism. If desired, colony counts as low as 10 CFU/ml may be determined after four hours of exposure to antimicrobics— by inoculating 0.1 ml of the broth cultures in addition to the 0.001-ml calibrated loopful. If, after overnight incubation, the four-hour colony counts do not clearly demonstrate antagonism or synergism, a 24-hour colony count might be appropriate, especially if the test organism is slow growing or if the broth is turbid in spite of a decreased colony count after four hours. With such a simplified approach, the evaluation of antimicrobic combinations by establishment of killing curves can be performed with relative ease in the average hospital laboratory.

Only time and experience will determine which of these two methods is more appropriate for determining whether a combination of antimicrobics is antagonistic or synergistic. There is a very real need for correlative studies of *in vitro* evaluations and *in vivo* effectiveness of antimicrobic combinations. Such data must be obtained before combination therapy can be placed upon a rational basis. The acceptance of standardized methods is essential before meaningful clinical trials can be carried out.

ENTEROCOCCAL RESISTANCE TO AMINOCYCLITOLS

By conventional criteria, enterococci are resistant to streptomycin (and other aminocyclitols) and are only moderately susceptible to the penicillins. However, many enterococci respond synergistically to the combination of these two types of antimicrobics and other strains do not display a synergistic effect. Figure 7-5 presents

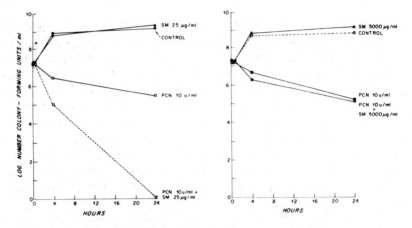

Figure 7-5. Effect of penicillin (PCN) and streptomycin (SM) singly and in combination against two enterococci, one moderately resistant to SM and the other highly resistant to SM. (From R. A. Zimmermann, R. C. Moellering, Jr., and A. N. Weinberg. 1971. J. Bacteriol. *105:* 875.)

the two types of killing curves that can be observed when enterococci are tested against streptomycin and benzylpenicillin.

Enterococci display one of two types of resistance to streptomycin. The first is a moderate degree of resistance (MIC = 62-500 μg/ml), which is the result of a relative impermeability of the cell to streptomycin. Antimicrobics such as the penicillins inhibit cell-wall synthesis, thus increasing the amount of streptomycin that may enter the individual cells. Once past this permeability barrier, streptomycin evokes extensive misreading or mistranslation of synthetic polynucleotide templates by the ribosomes within such moderately resistant cells. The second type of resistance is a high-level resistance (MIC $\geqslant$ 2,000 μg/ml). Although cell wall–inhibiting antimicrobics increase the amount of streptomycin entering such highly resistant cells, the ribosomes are not affected. For that reason, such microorganisms fail to respond synergistically to a combination of streptomycin and penicillin.[17,18]

Moellering et al.[13,14] proposed a simple screening test for predicting the presence or absence of synergism between penicillin and one or more of the aminocyclitols. Enterococci are screened for high-level resistance to streptomycin, kanamycin, or gentamicin by the streaking of a colony onto drug-containing nutrient agar plates (dextrose-phosphate broth with 0.8% agar). Four plates are inoculated—one a control without antimicrobics and the others containing different aminocyclitols at a concentration of 2,000 μg/ml. After overnight incubation at 35°C, the plates are examined for clear evidence of growth. Those enterococci that show no growth or, at most, a slight haziness at the origin of the streaking but yet show viability on the control plate are likely to respond favorably to the combination of antimicrobics. Enterococci that produce a few isolated colonies or confluent growth are highly resistant to the aminocyclitol, and therefore the addition of penicillin is not likely to be synergistic. Such high-level resistance to streptomycin is fairly common among clinical isolates of enterococci and thus strains could be tested before combined therapy is initiated. The simple screening test for high-level resistance might provide extremely valuable information before the more cumbersome direct test of synergism can be completed.

REFERENCES

1. Barry, A. L., and L. D. Sabath. 1974. Special tests: Bactericidal activity and activity of antimicrobics in combination. In *Manual of Clinical Microbiology.* 2d ed. E. H. Lennette, E. H. Spaulding, and J. P. Truant (Eds.). American Society for Microbiology, Washington, D. C. pp. 431-435.
2. Bulger, R. J., and K. Nielson. 1968. Effect of different media on *in vitro* studies of antibiotic combinations. Appl. Microbiol. *16:*890-895.
3. Chabbert, Y. A., and J. C. Patte. 1960. Cellophane transfer: Application to the study of activity of combination of antibiotics. Appl. Microbiol. *8:* 193-199.
4. Dye, W. E. 1956. An agar diffusion method for studying the bacteriostatic action of combinations of antimicrobial agents. In *Antibiotics Annual 1955-1956.* Medical Encyclopedia, Inc., pp. 374-382.
5. Elion, G. B., S. Singer, and G. H. Hitchings. 1954. Antagonists of nucleic acid derivatives VII. Synergism in combination of biochemically related antimetabolites. J. Biol. Chem. *208:* 477-488.
6. Garrod, L. P., and P. M. Waterworth. 1962. Methods of testing combined antibiotic bactericidal action and the significance of the results. J. Clin. Pathol. *15:* 328-338.
7. Hoeprich, P. D. 1972. Antimicrobics and antihelmintics for systemic therapy. In *Infectious Diseases.* P. D. Hoeprich (Ed.). Harper & Row, Hagerstown, Maryland. pp. 177-206.
8. Jawetz, E., and J. B. Gunnison. 1952. Studies on antibiotic synergism and antagonism: A scheme of combined antibiotic action. Antibiot. Chemother. *2:* 243-248.
9. Jawetz, E., J. B. Gunnison, and U. R. Coleman. 1954. Observations on the mode of action of antibiotic synergism and antagonism. J. Gen. Microbiol. *10:* 191-198.
10. Jawetz, E., and M. Sonne. 1966. Penicillin-streptomycin treatment of enterococcal endocarditis: A re-evaluation. N. Engl. J. Med. *274:* 710-715.
11. Lee, W. S., and L. Komarmy. 1975. Simple technique for the assay of antibiotic synergism against enterococci. Antimicrob. Agents Chemother. *7:* 82-84.
12. Lorian, V., and G. Fodor. 1974. Technique for determining the bactericidal effect of drug combinations. Antimicrob. Agents Chemother. *5:* 630-633.
13. Moellering, R., A. Weinberg, R. Zimmermann, and C. Wennersten. 1970. Antibiotic synergism against group D streptococci. Clin. Res. *18:* 445.
14. Moellering, R. C., C. Wennersten, T. Medrek, and A. N. Weinberg. 1971. Prevalence of high-level resistance to aminoglycosides in clinical isolates of enterococci. Antimicrob. Agents Chemother.-1970, pp. 335-340.
15. Sabath, L. D. 1968. Synergy of antibacterial substances by apparently known mechanisms. Antimicrob. Agents Chemother.-1967, pp. 210-217.

16. Stokes, E. J. 1968. *Clinical Bacteriology*. 3rd ed. Williams & Wilkins, Baltimore. pp. 170-216.
17. Zimmermann, R. A., R. C. Moellering, Jr., and A. N. Weinberg. 1971. Enterococcal resistance to antibiotic synergism. Antimicrob. Agents Chemother.-1970, pp. 517-521.
18. Zimmermann, R. A., R. C. Moellering, Jr., and A. N. Weinberg. 1971. Mechanism of resistance to antibiotic synergism in enterococci. J. Bacteriol. *105:* 873-879.

Chapter 8

ANTIMICROBIC DILUTION TESTS: QUALITY CONTROL AND TROUBLESHOOTING

Quality control actually means much more than simply testing a standard control strain frequently enough to be sure that all is going well. Quality control is best thought of as a formalized program consisting of a series of procedures each selected to monitor one or more specific sources of error. When a control procedure indicates a possible problem, a positive plan of action should be available for troubleshooting and correcting the faulty technique. There should be enough controls to allow one to pinpoint the source of the difficulty when the test procedure is found to be performing unsatisfactorily.

Since each laboratory situation is somewhat different, the quality-control program has to be individualized. For obvious reasons a laboratory routinely testing clinical isolates by a dilution technique needs a quality-control program that differs significantly from that required to control a well-defined study comparing two or more drugs. The relative importance of different sources of error depends upon whether agar or broth dilution techniques are being applied, as well as on the type of antimicrobics and kind of mi-

117

croorganism being tested. Awareness of the specific problems inherent in the type of test system being controlled is essential for developing a meaningful quality-control program. For optimal results, it is necessary to develop a rational balance between the amount of effort required for each control procedure, the frequency with which a particular source of error may occur, and the seriousness of the potential error, that is, the likelihood of a clinically important misinterpretation.

The principles of quality-control procedures for antimicrobic dilution techniques can be defined best by first considering the more common sources of error that need to be controlled. Special problems arising from tests with specific antimicrobics or groups of microorganisms should also be considered from the point of view of quality control. The general steps that can be taken to control these potential sources of error can then be outlined in broad terms. This type of information may be synthesized to develop a meaningful control program for each individual laboratory situation.

COMMON SOURCES OF ERROR

1. Errors in Preparation and Storage of Stock Solutions
   a. Simple errors in arithmetic
   b. Inappropriate standard powers or solutions
   c. Inadequate solvent or diluent
   d. Improper storage conditions

2. Errors in Preparing Antimicrobic Dilutions
   a. Errors in calculating dilution schedule
   b. Volumetric errors in pipetting
   c. Mechanical failure of semi-automated diluting systems
   d. Failure to cool agar medium before adding drugs
   e. Inappropriate storage of agar plates or microdilution trays

3. Errors Involving the Test Medium
   a. Deviation from the standard medium without adequate controls
   b. Failure to check pH and cation content
   c. Medium nutritionally inadequate for the strain being tested
   d. Failure to detect contamination of medium
   e. Inappropriate storage of medium before use

4. Standardization of Inoculum with a $BaSO_4$ Turbidity Standard
   a. Carelessness in adjusting broth cultures
   b. Inappropriately prepared turbidity standard
   c. Failure to check and replace turbidity standard periodically
   d. Variability resulting in cell mass or growth phase of the strains being tested

5. Standardization of Inoculum by Dilution of Stationary-Phase Broth Cultures
   a. Attempts to apply this approach to tests with slow-growing fastidious microorganisms
   b. Use with strains tha fail to produce a uniform turbidity in the broth medium
   c. Failure to mix broth cultures thoroughly on vortex mixer
   d. Inadequate control of incubation time and temperature
   e. Inadequate inoculum to initiate rapid growth
   f. Errors in dilution of broth cultures

6. Errors Occurring during Inoculation of Tests
    a. Mechanical failure or misuse of inoculum replicators, resulting in skipped tubes or plates
    b. Inaccuracy and imprecision of inoculating apparatus
    c. Improper care of inoculum replicators
    d. Failure to isolate swarming *Proteus* sp. on agar dilution plates
    e. Inadequate drying of agar surface before inoculation
    f. Inversion of inoculated agar plates before inoculum spots have absorbed

7. Errors Involving Incubation of the Tests
    a. Failure to control incubator temperature
    b. Inattention to location of plates or trays on incubator racks (height of stacks)
    c. Improper control of incubation time
    d. Incubation under increased CO_2 or anaerobic atmosphere without adequate control

8. Errors in Reading and Reporting Test Results
    a. Improper controls to detect contamination or tests with mixed cultures
    b. Variability inherent in reading "soft" end-points
    c. Clerical errors in transposing data.

The above list of potential sources of error may be used as a checklist for troubleshooting the broth or agar dilution procedure when the tests are out of control. The relative importance of such sources of error depends somewhat upon the type of antimicrobic agent and general type of microorganism being tested. If a battery of antimicrobic agents is being tested against the same microorganism, certain variables may influence the results obtained with some antimicrobics much more than those obtained with other antimicrobics, and thus it is often possible to identify the most likely source of the problem according to the type of antimicrobics showing a decreased precision or accuracy.

PROBLEMS COMMON TO SPECIFIC TYPES OF ANTIMICROBIC AGENTS

Penicillins. Most penicillins are relatively unstable in solution at temperatures above freezing, and many are especially sensitive to inactivation in acid solutions. Hydrolysis of benzylpenicillin results in the production of penicilloic acid, thus lowering the pH and, in turn, accelerating further deterioration of the drug. For that reason, concentrated solutions are less stable than dilute solutions. In a medium with a fermentable carbohydrate, a decrease in pH might occur as a result of early microbial metabolism. The amount of active penicillin could be decreased enough to result in secondary overgrowth of otherwise susceptible microorganisms. When testing microorganisms that produce a penicillin-inactivating enzyme, the inoculum density is extremely critical and must be controlled carefully.

Cephalosporins. Most cephalosporins are relatively unstable in solutions at temperatures above freezing. At normal incubation temperature, cephalothin is inactivated fairly rapidly, so that by 12 hours, about half of the initial concentration remains biologically active, thus permitting secondary overgrowth of any remaining viable microorganisms. For that reason, susceptible strains may appear to be resistant at the end of a standard 24-hour incubation period but susceptible after 12 hours of incubation.[14] Some microorganisms also produce a cephalosporinase that is responsible for additional degradation of the cephalosporins. In testing such strains, the density of inoculum is particularly important and must be defined carefully.

Aminocyclitols. Generally, the activity of aminocyclitols is increased at an alkaline pH and decreased under acidic conditions. *In vitro* activity is markedly influenced by the concentration of various inorganic ions in the medium.[5,11] Increased concentrations of NaCl can reduce the activity of most aminocyclitols. Various divalent cations, especially Ca^{++} and Mg^{++}, decrease the activity of these drugs, the effect being particularly profound when testing *Pseudomonas aeruginosa*. With *P. aeruginosa*, broth dilution MICs are significantly lower than those obtained by agar dilution because of the additional divalent cations contributed to the medium by the agar itself.

Polypeptides. Both colistin and polymyxin B are fairly stable in solution but rapidly inactivated in alkaline conditions (pH above 8). Inactivation by various inorganic substances that can contaminate unwashed agar has been reported.[7,8,10] Increasing the concentration of divalent cations also decreases the activity of the polypeptides.

Tetracyclines. Most tetracyclines are reasonably stable in solution, but chlortetracycline is extremely unstable. In nutrient broth at pH 7.4, chlortetracycline loses most of its activity during overnight incubation, whereas tetracycline HCl loses 10% to 20% of its activity. Free divalent cations in the medium decrease the activity of tetracycline by chelation of the antibiotic, and thus the test medium must be controlled to avoid variable results.

Macrolides. Erythromycin is fairly stable in slightly alkaline solutions, but activity is lost rapidly at pH below 6. *In vitro* activity is markedly affected by the pH; it is most active at a pH of 8.5 and much less active at a pH of 6. Incubation under increased CO_2 atmosphere decreases the pH enough to reduce the activity of erythromycin.

Sulfonamides. *In vitro* susceptibility tests with the sulfonamides can be very misleading. Use of a light inoculum is extremely important.[2] Traces of *p*-aminobenzoic acid, methionine, or other amino acids and purines in the test medium competitively inhibit the sulfonamides. Addition of lysed horse blood neutralizes the effect of such inhibitors.[3] Traces of inhibitors carried over in the inoculum or included in the test medium may permit initial growth of the microorganism for a few generations, with eventual growth inhibition once the drug inhibitors are depleted. As a result, the end-points may be "fuzzy," and a faint film of growth seen on plates beyond an otherwise obvious end-point could be misinterpreted as indicating resistance. As a general rule, the appropriate end-point may be taken as that concentration that results in inhibition of at least 80% of the growth seen on the control plates. With an appropriate test medium and light inoculum, the end-points should be easily discerned.

Trimethoprim. This potential inhibitor of dihydrofolate reductase is active *in vitro*, but the *in vitro* inhibitory activity is inversely correlated with the amount of thymidine in the test medium.[3] Each batch of medium should be tested for absence of trimethoprim antagonists before *in vitro* tests are carried out. Enterococci are particularly sensitive to the antagonistic effect resulting from trace amounts of thymidine in the test medium.

SELECTION AND USE OF STANDARD CONTROL STRAINS

The precision and accuracy of the test procedure can be monitored by including a standard control organism of known susceptibility each time a batch of tests is performed. The control organism may represent one of the standard control strains designated for the disc diffusion technique ("Seattle" *Staphylococcus aureus* and *Escherichia coli* or the "Boston" *Pseudomonas aeruginosa*), or it may be an isolate recovered within an individual laboratory and carried in stock culture for control purposes. The ideal control strain should have the following characteristics:

1. Stability upon long-term storage is an essential characteristic of any quality-control strain. As a general rule, resistant mutants are not stable enough and thus strains selected from the normally susceptible population for a given genus are preferred.
2. The MIC should be within the range of concentrations being tested. Potentially useful control strains should include representatives from different species that normally display MICs within the range of concentrations being tested for each antimicrobic.
3. The test strain must be capable of growing adequately in the standard medium, without further supplementation of the medium.
4. The control test should display sharply defined end-points and thus reproducible results when the test is "in control."

5. When specific antagonists in the medium are known to influence the antimicrobic being tested, the control strain should be one that is known to be susceptible to
fairly minor changes in the test medium. For example, a strain of *P. aeruginosa*
should be included in the battery of cultures useful for controlling tests with gentamicin because of its unique susceptibility to minor changes in the concentration of
magnesium and calcium.[11]

To avoid variation and contamination, the control strain should
not be subcultured repeatedly on slants or in broth. Appropriate
control strains can be maintained lyophilized, frozen at –60°C in
suitably stabilized media, such as skim milk, 15% glycerol broth, or
50% inactivated fetal calf serum in broth, or they may be purchased
from a laboratory supply house as single-use vials specifically developed for quality-control purposes.

The following method has been found to be a convenient way to
maintain those control strains that are tested on a regular basis.[1]
Once a year, a lyophilized sample is reconstituted and transferred
to a blood or chocolate agar plate. A very dense suspension of colonies is then prepared in trypticase soy broth without glucose and
with 15% glycerol added. This cell suspension is divided into 12
samples of from 1 to 2 ml each and stored at –60°C. The first of each
month a frozen sample is thawed and subcultured onto a blood or
chocolate plate; after overnight incubation, from five to ten colonies are transferred to a trypticase soy agar slant (with blood or
other supplements required for growth of the control strain). After
overnight incubation, the slant is stored in a refrigerator for the rest
of the week. Once a week, growth from the agar slant is transferred
to a blood agar or chocolate agar plate and five to ten colonies
from the subculture are transferred to another agar slant. All culture
tests are initiated with five to ten colonies selected from a
fresh agar plate subculture—never from the stored agar slant directly, and slants are never held more than one week. Experience has
emphasized the need for meticulous care of the stock cultures before it is possible to pinpoint the source of the difficulty when the
test is "out of control." The system of storage of stock cultures
described above is only one approach; it has proven to be practical
and requires a minimum of effort. Those laboratories not having
access to a –60°C freezer might have equal success in storing most
control strains at –20°C in glycerol broth for as long as one year.

GENERAL PRINCIPLES OF QUALITY CONTROL

A well-organized system for carrying out each step of the standard procedure is essential to a successful testing program. As with
most laboratory procedures, dependable results can be obtained
only when the techniques are used on a regular basis. When done

infrequently, extensive controls must be included with each test, whereas fewer controls are needed once a well-organized testing program has been established.

The system for storing standard drugs and stock solutions is critically important, especially with the less stable penicillins and cephalosporins. Most errors occur as a result of simple mistakes in arithmetic, and thus all calculations should be double-checked by a second person before stock solutions are prepared or diluted. Standard control strains must be tested to monitor the overall accuracy and precision of the testing procedure; the results with such controls determine whether such common problems are being encountered.

Interpretation of Tests with Control Strains. To control accuracy of the diluted technique, the "true" MIC value for each antimicrobic should be known for each control strain. Unfortunately, the absolute MIC value for a given strain is too method-dependent to permit an unqualified definition of the control limits for a given strain. Until universally accepted standard methods are available, each laboratory should establish its own control values (as defined in Table 8-1 for a microdilution technique) by repeated testing of the control strain with the particular technique being used. In gen-

Table 8-1. **Microdilution MIC Values Normally Obtained with Two Control Strains Tested in Mueller-Hinton Broth without Added Cations**

	"Seattle" *E. coli*	"Portland" *S. faecalis*
Ampicillin	4.0	1.0
Carbenicillin	8.0	32
Cephalothin	8.0	16.0
Chloramphenicol	4.0	4.0
Gentamicin	0.5	8.0
Kanamycin	2.0	32
Polymyxin B	0.5	> 8.0
Tetracycline	1.0	>16
Nitrofurantoin	8.0	16
Clindamycin	>16	8.0
Erythromycin	>16	2.0
Nafcillin	> 8	4.0
Penicillin G	> 4	2.0

SOURCE: C. Riedel. Micro-Media Systems, Inc., Palo Alto, Calif. Unpublished data. (Table based on tests with approximately 30 different lots of micro-dilution trays.)

eral, the MIC values should vary no more than one doubling dilution above or below the mode, and with well-controlled procedures the MICs should be within one dilution step on either side of the geometric mean. The control strains should be included with each batch of tests, and the modal and/or geometric mean MIC periodically recalculated as experience is gained with each antimicrobic. A sudden deviation from the norm indicates that the test is "out of control" and suggests that the test results may not be valid. In this way the controls are at least monitoring the precision of the testing procedure if not controlling the accuracy of the antimicrobic dilutions.

Control of Individual Test Strains. When it is necessary to deviate from the standard procedure in order to test fastidious or slow-growing microorganisms, the control strains are invaluable. They can be used to determine whether an alteration in procedure (e.g., supplementation of the test medium, extension of the incubation period, utilization of increased CO_2 atmospheres) significantly affects the test results.

Even if the control strains indicate acceptable results, there is no absolute guarantee that the test microorganism was properly standardized and the plates or tubes properly inoculated. Purity of each test strain should be checked, especially if a broth dilution technique is being used. A simple disc diffusion test is an excellent way to detect a minor population of resistant variants or contaminants in the initial inoculum. With the agar dilution technique, careful examination of the test plates at or near the end-point often reveals such mixed cultures. The density of inoculum actually achieved should be checked periodically by preparing a simple dilution of the adjusted inoculum and then streaking a nutrient agar plate with a calibrated loop. Such controls are particularly important when testing antimicrobics that are especially affected by variations in the inoculum density. Since it is not always possible to check every test strain, periodic spot checks should be carried out as often as is practical.

Finally, experience with a given antimicrobic and selected species of microorganisms permits one to establish the range of MICs normally seen. Those strains that display MICs far above or below this normal range should be re-examined carefully to rule out the possibility of technical error. A review of laboratory records can establish the values being obtained with selected species and antimicrobics in order to detect gradual changes in technique or to compare results of tests in different laboratories using similar methods. With the aid of a computerized system, it is possible to

establish formally the range of MICs normally seen with susceptible strains of a given species for each antimicrobic, thus identifying
those strains that require further examination before being reported.

In short, a doubting mind—one that appreciates the many
sources of error—a cautious attitude, and experience may be combined to detect errors that are otherwise unidentified with the
usual quality-control procedures.

REFERENCES

1. Barry, A. L., G. D. Fay, and F. W. Atchison. 1972. Quality control of antimicrobial disc susceptibility testing with a rapid method compared to the standard
   methods. Antimicrob. Agents Chemother. 2: 419-422.
2. Bauer, A. W., and J. C. Sherris. 1964. The determination of sulfonamide susceptibility of bacteria. Chemotherapia 9: 1-19.
3. Ferone, R., S. R. M. Bushby, J. J. Burchall, W. D. Moore, and D. Smith. 1975.
   Identification of Harper-Cawston factor as thymidine phosphorylase and removal from media of substances interfering with susceptibility testing to sulfonamides and diaminopyrimidines. Antimicrob. Agents Chemother. 7: 91-98.
4. Garrod, L. P., H. P. Lambert, and F. O'Grady (with a chapter on laboratory
   methods by P. M. Waterworth). 1973. *Antibiotic and Chemotherapy*, 4th ed.
   Churchill Livingstone, Edinburgh.
5. Garrod, L. P., and P. M. Waterworth. 1969. Effect of medium composition on
   the apparent sensitivity of *Pseudomonas aeruginosa* to gentamicin. J. Clin.
   Pathol. 22: 534-538.
6. Goodman, L. S., and A. Gilman. 1970. *The Pharmacological Basis of Therapeutics*, 4th ed. Macmillan, New York.
7. Hanus, F. J., J. G. Sands, and E. O. Bennett. 1967. Antibiotic activity in the
   presence of agar. Appl. Microbiol. 15: 31-34.
8. Kunin, C. M., and W. P. Edmondson. 1968. Inhibitor of antibiotics in bac-
   teriologic agar. Proc. Soc. Exp. Biol. Med. 129: 118-122.
9. Lorian, V. 1966. *Antibiotics and Chemotherapeutic Agents in Clinical and
   Laboratory Practice*. Charles C Thomas, Springfield, Ill.
10. Newton, B. A. 1953. Reversal of the antibacterial activity of polymyxin by diva-
    lent cations. Nature 172: 160-161.
11. Reller, L. B., F. D. Schoenknecht, M. A. Kenny, and J. C. Sherris. 1974. Antibio-
    tic susceptibility testing of *Pseudomonas aeruginosa*: Selection of a control
    strain and criteria for magnesium and calcium content of media. J. Infect. Dis.
    130: 454-463.
12. Ryan, K. J., G. M. Needham, C. L. Dunsmoor, and J. C. Sherris. 1970. Stability
    of antibiotics and chemotherapeutics in agar plates. Appl. Microbiol. 20: 447-
    451.
13. Vera, H. D., and M. Dumoff. 1974. Culture media. In *Manual of Clinical Mi-
    crobiology*, 2d ed. E. H. Lennette, E. H. Spaulding, and J. P. Truant (Eds.).
    American Society for Microbiology, Washington, D. C. pp.879-929.
14. Wick, W. E. 1964. Influence of antibiotic stability on the results of *in vitro*
    testing procedures. J. Bacteriol. 87: 1162-1170.

Section III
SPECIAL TEST
PROCEDURES

Chapter 9

DETECTION OF STAPHYLOCOCCAL PENICILLIN β-LACTAMASE ACTIVITY

Microorganisms produce a large variety of enzymes, some of which are capable of inactivating antimicrobial agents. Those enzymes that inactivate the penicillins are referred to generically as penicillinases, those that inactivate the cephalosporins are called cephalosporinases. They may also be classified according to their site of action, e.g., β-lactamase and amidase (Fig. 9-1). Such enzymes are most precisely referred to by specifying both the substrate (antimicrobic) and the site of action, e.g., penicillin β-lactamase.

GENERAL CHARACTERISTICS OF PENICILLIN β-LACTAMASE

All penicillin-resistant strains of *Staphylococcus aureus* found in clinical material are capable of producing a penicillin β-lactamase that hydrolyzes the amide bond in the β-lactam ring of 6-amino penicillinic acid with the production of the biologically inactive penicilloic acid. Although the bacterial cells are susceptible to the inhibitory action of penicillin, they are resistant by virtue of their ability to produce penicillinase, which is capable of inactivating

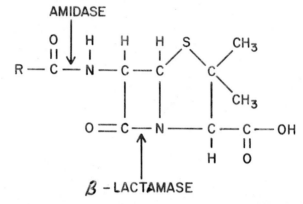

Figure 9-1.   Site of action of penicillin β-lactamase and penicillin amidase on the penicillin molecule.

the drug before it can exert its lethal effect. Susceptible strains of *S. aureus* do not produce penicillinase enzymes. For that reason, a test that determines the capacity to produce penicillinase should predict penicillin resistance accurately—and better than an MIC determination, which could be misleadingly low if a light inoculum were used.

Although much of the penicillin β-lactamase enzyme is firmly bound to the cell, a certain proportion is found free in the surrounding medium. The amount of extracellular enzyme is determined largely by the environmental conditions, which determine whether the penicillinase remains ionically bound to the cell. The anionic content and pH of the medium determine to a great extent the amount of extracellular enzyme.

Although a certain amount of β-lactamase is constitutive, the production of additional enzyme may be induced by almost any compound that contains a β-lactam ring. The kinetics of staphylococcal penicillinase induction depends upon the properties of the inducer and on the ionic composition and pH of the medium, as well as on the particular strain being studied. Although most penicillins and cephalosporins are capable of inducing the production of penicillin β-lactamase, some are more active inducers than others. The so-called penicillinase-resistant penicillins and the cephalosporins are excellent inducers of staphylococcal penicillinase although they are relatively resistant to hydrolysis by the enzyme, possibly because their β-lactam ring is somehow protected by the spatial arrangement of the additional radicals attached to the molecule.

Penicillin β-lactamase can be assayed quantitatively or detected qualitatively by a variety of methods. Results of quantitative tests depend upon a number of contributing factors, such as the presence of contaminating enzymes, location and degree of binding of the enzyme within the cell, the inducible expression of the enzyme loss of activity by dilution, inactivation by reagents used in the assay, and choice of the appropriate substrate. β-lactamase activity is usually detected by indirectly measuring the product, penicilloic acid, by one of several iodometric methods or by detecting the increased acidity that occurs as the acidic product accumulates.

RAPID QUALITATIVE TESTS

Penicillin is the most desirable therapeutic agent for treatment of infections caused by susceptible strains of *S. aureus*. A penicillinase-resistant penicillin is much more expensive and less efficient but necessary for treatment of infections caused by strains capable of producing a penicillin β-lactamase. A rapid method for qualitatively detecting the capacity of individual isolates to produce penicillinase would be useful in guiding the proper choice of antimicrobic therapy. The following simple methods have been proposed for quick identification of penicillin resistance among isolates of *S. aureus* from clinical specimens.

Iodometric Methods. Penicilloic acid binds iodine, removing the blue color of an iodine-starch mixture. Individual colonies may be tested in one of two ways, according to the methods of Foley and Perret.[4]

1. A single colony may be removed from the surface of a primary agar plate culture and emulsified in 0.2 ml of a solution containing 10,000 units of penicillin G per ml in 0.05 M phosphate buffer (pH 6.5). After one hour at room temperature one drop of a starch-iodine solution (equal parts of 1% sodium starch glycolate and 0.04 N iodine) is mixed with the test suspension. Decolorization proceeds rapidly with most penicillinase-producing strains. The test is considered positive if all color disappears within five minutes and negative if the blue color remains after five minutes.

2. Whatman No. 1 filter paper that has been impregnated with fresh 1% starch solution and dried and cut into strips is dipped into a solution of penicillin G (10,000 units/ml in 0.05 M phosphate buffer), drained, and laid carefully over the colony to be tested so as to exclude air bubbles. After 30 minutes at room temperature, 1 ml of a 0.04 N iodine solution is added directly to the filter-paper strip. Within 30 minutes, the filter paper above penicillinase-producing colonies develops a white color but the paper over nonproducers of penicillinase remains blue as a result of the iodine-starch reaction.

Methicillin-Induced PNCB Tests. Novick's PNCB reagent (N-phenyl-l-naphthylamine-azo-o-carboxybenzene) is an acid-base indicator that is water soluble and orange-yellow when basic and water insoluble and deep purple when acid.[5] With the production of penicilloic acid, another –COOH group is added to each penicillin molecule and thus the pH decreases enough to change the indicator from its soluble basic form to the water-insoluble purple compound. This reagent has been used for the detection of staphylococcal penicillinase after induction by methicillin or other lactam antibiotics.

1. The methicillin-induced PNCB test of Duma and Kunz[3] first requires a standard agar diffusion disc susceptibility test with a 5-μg methicillin disc. After overnight incubation, growth at the edge of the zone of inhibition will have been exposed to concentrations of methicillin that are maximal for induction of the β-lactamase. The susceptibility plates are opened and dried at 35°C for one hour. Next, the area of growth proximal to the zone of inhibition is flooded with 1.5 ml of a 0.25% (w/v) stock solution of PNCB dissolved in N, N-dimethylformamide with 6% (v/v) 1 N NaOH. The plates are then allowed to dry 45 minutes under a hood. After drying, the areas stained by the PNCB indicator are flooded with 1.5 ml of a refrigerated stock solution of 10% (w/v) aqueous potassium penicillin G. If penicillinase is present, a purple precipitate will form over the colonies just outside the zone of inhibition. The staphylococcus is considered a nonproducer of penicillinase if no color change is seen after 45 minutes.

This technique has been simplified by Adams, Barry, and Benner.[2] The drying time is reduced by incorporating the PNCB reagent into a melted and cooled (50°C) 1.5% aqueous agar solution (1 ml in 4 ml of agar, or 1 ml in 8 ml of agar, depending on the size of petri plates tested). The solution is mixed and spread as a thin agar overlay that quickly solidifies enough to permit flooding with the penicillin solution. This procedure is particularly useful for testing strains that give penicillin zones in the intermediate, equivocal range (21–28 mm). Such "no decision" test results can be resolved easily in less than an hour. Nafcillin, oxacillin, methicillin, and cephalothin discs have been found to be satisfactory inducers of penicillinase, but they should be located adjacent to penicillin, ampicillin, or other lactam drugs since other antimicrobics may interfere with the induction of penicillinase if the discs are too close to the inducer.

2. A rapid methicillin-induced PNCB test has been also described by Adams et al.[2] to permit rapid testing of fresh clinical isolates. From one to five colonies are transferred to a Mueller-Hinton agar plate so as to yield a band of confluent growth. A 1-μg oxacillin (or a 5-μg methicillin) disc is placed on one end of the inoculated area and a 30-μg cephalothin disc is applied to the other end. After four to five hours at 35°C, staphylococcal growth becomes visible and induction of penicillinase can be detected with the procedure described above.

Direct Capillary Tube Method. An even simpler direct method for detecting staphylococcal penicillinase in non-induced primary isolates has been described by Rosen, Jacobson, and Rudderman.[6] This technique may be used also to test samples of induced growth on a susceptibility plate when the penicillin zones are indeterminant. Furthermore, Thornsberry and Kirven[7] have reported success in using this technique for screening non-induced colonies of type B *Hemophilus influenzae* in order to distinguish between ampicillin-resistant and ampicillin-susceptible strains.

In this procedure, a large mass of bacterial growth is exposed to a solution of penicillin with a phenol red indicator, within the narrow confines of a capillary tube. The production of penicilloic acid is detected by the color change that results from the decreased pH. The test solution is prepared by adding 16.6 ml of water and 2 ml of a 0.5% phenol red solution to a vial containing 20 million units of penicillin G (buffered potassium penicillin G for injection). Sodium hydroxide (1 M) is added in drops until the solution just turns violet (pH 8.5). This penicillin solution may be divided into 1-ml aliquots and stored as long as one week at –20°C. Thawed tubes may be kept at 4°C for an entire working day, but longer storage is not advisable because of the possible hydrolysis of penicillin. As penicillin is hydrolyzed, the color of the solution changes from violet or deep red to yellow (acidic form); such stock solutions should be discarded as soon as a yellow color begins to appear.

To perform the rapid capillary tube test, the penicillin test solution is allowed to run into a capillary tube (0.5 to 0.9 mm ID) and the fluid is allowed to flow by capillary action to a distance of from 1 to 2 cm. The tip of the capillary tube is then scraped across a colony to be tested, care being taken to avoid entrapment of air between the test solution and the plug of bacteria, which should fill the bottom of the tube. The filled capillary tubes are then allowed to incubate at room temperature in a vertical position. This may be achieved by sticking the empty end of the capillary tube into clay and letting it hang straight down. If the organisms contain β-lactamase, the bacterial plug will turn yellow within one hour. By that time, the test solution above the bacterial plug usually turns yellow as well.

REFERENCES

1. Abramson, C. 1972. Staphylococcal enzymes. In *The Staphylococci*. J. O. Cohen (Ed.). Wiley-Interscience, New York. pp. 187-248.
2. Adams, A. P., A. L. Barry, and E. J. Benner. 1970. A simple, rapid test to differentiate penicillin-susceptible from penicillin-resistant *Staphylococcus aureus*. J. Infect. Dis. *122:* 544-546.
3. Duma, R. J., and L. J. Kunz. 1968. Simple test for identifying penicillinase-producing staphylococci. Appl. Microbiol. *16:* 1261-1262.
4. Foley, J. M., and C. J. Perret. 1962. Screening bacterial colonies for penicillinase production. Nature *195:* 287-288.
5. Novick, R. P., and M. H. Richmond. 1965. Nature and interaction of the genetic elements governing penicillinase synthesis in *Staphylococcus aureus*. J. Bacteriol. *90:* 467-480.
6. Rosen, I. G., J. Jacobson, and R. Rudderman. 1972. Rapid capillary tube method for detecting penicillin resistance in *Staphylococcus aureus*. Appl. Microbiol. *23:* 649-650.
7. Thornsberry, C., and L. A. Kirven. 1974. Ampicillin resistance in *Hemophilus influenzae* as determined by a rapid test for beta-lactamase production. Antimicrob. Agents Chemother. *6:* 653-654.

Chapter 10

A SEMI-AUTOMATED DISC
ELUTION TEST SYSTEM

The development of automated or semi-automated systems for performing susceptibility tests is likely to provide not only a greater efficiency and convenience but also a greater uniformity of results by virtue of the fact that instrumentation requires an objective definition of each step in the testing procedure, including those manipulations that are rather subjectively performed with the currently available manual methods, e.g., standardization of inoculum and determination of end-points. Finally, most mechanized readout systems are easily adapted for direct input into computerized data processing systems, thus permitting direct reporting of the test results and storage of data for later analysis.

With automation, relatively sophisticated measurements can be applied to determine the early response of a microorganism to the antimicrobial agent, thus opening the potential for a truly rapid test system. Such early readings may not correlate completely with results of more orthodox tests since some microorganisms respond to sub-inhibitory concentrations of an antimicrobic, with a prolonged lag phase, or initial reduction in viable cells, with eventual overgrowth. For that reason, early readings might indicate susceptibility, whereas the more conventional determinations made after overnight incubation suggest resistance. When the secondary over-growth occurs as a result of antimicrobic deterioration, the early readings might be more appropriate, but when the delayed response represents growth of a resistant variant selected *in vitro* by the sub-inhibitory concentration of antimicrobic, the early test results might be misleading. As further experience is gained with automated rapid test systems and discrepancies with the more conventional test systems are better documented, it will be necessary to maintain an open-minded attitude toward the possibility that the newer methods might actually be providing a better estimate of clinical responsiveness or nonresponsiveness.

The Autobac I system (Fig. 10-1) represents one such instrumental approach toward the goal of automated rapid susceptibility testing.[3] This test system has been subjected to rather extensive preliminary evaluation[2] and has withstood a rather rigorous evaluation

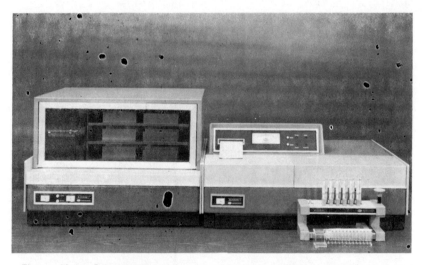

Figure 10-1. Components of Autobac 1 instrument system. *Right foreground*: 13-chamber cuvette and disc dispenser; *right background*: light-scattering photometer; *left background*: separate incubator/shaker.

"in the field."[4] For these reasons, the test system is described in some detail in the following pages—as an example of what can be accomplished with relatively simple instrumentation. Other systems using slightly different approaches are currently being developed, but they have not yet been sufficiently evaluated for marketing in this country. The Autobac I system encompasses the principle of a disc elution broth technique in which the drug is carried to the test medium in the form of a filter-paper disc containing a fixed amount of antimicrobic, thus providing a known concentration of drug with a minimum amount of time and effort on the part of the operator. After a short period of time at an appropriate temperature, growth of the microorganism is detected by measuring the amount of light scattered from the bacterial suspension.

AUTOBAC I TEST SYSTEM

The Autobac I system (Pfizer Diagnostics, New York) consists of four basic components, as shown in Figures 10-1 and 10-2.

1. A disposable 13-chamber cuvette, which contains a means of conveniently distributing a broth inoculum to 13 testing chambers and suspending antibiotic "elution discs" in 12 of these chambers (Figs. 10-2 and 10-3).

2. A disc dispenser, which loads the cuvette with a panel of 12 antimicrobial agents (Fig. 10-1, foreground).

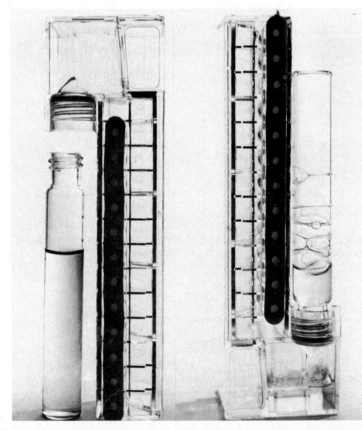

Figure 10-2. Autobac cuvettes. Inoculated broth is diluted after adjusting turbidity, and the tube is then screwed into a cuvette (*left*), which is then inverted to fill the reservoir (*right*).

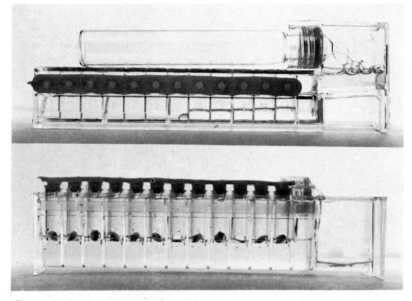

Figure 10-3. Cuvette chambers. The cuvette is turned horizontally to fill the rear channel (*top*), and the cuvette is then rotated to fill each of the 13 separate chambers (*bottom*).

3. A 36°C incubator/shaker, which agitates the cuvette contents for the three-to five-hour incubation period, employing a ¾ inch amplitude rotary motion at 220 rpm. Each incubator holds as many as 30 cuvettes at one time; additional incubators may be added to handle more tests.

4. A photometer, which automatically scans each chamber of the cuvette, measures the amount of light scattered from the bacterial suspension, and prints the results. The photometer is used also to standardize the density of the initial inoculum.

Test Procedure. Morphologically similar colonies are picked from the initial culture and suspended in 6 ml of a buffered saline solution. The saline tube is then inserted into the instrument and the inoculum concentration adjusted to between 1 and 2 $\times$ 10^7 organisms per ml and then diluted in Eugonic broth (Pfizer) for a final inoculum concentration of 10^6 organisms per ml. The inoculated broth tube is then screwed into the cuvette, into which a panel of elution test discs has already been added. The assembly is inverted so that the broth flows into the cuvette reservoir. The cuvette is then rotated 90 degrees to its back surface so that the inoculum flows in the rear channel across the cuvette. A final rotation to the upright position places equal aliquots of inoculated broth in each measured chamber. The cuvette is then placed in the incubator/shaker and incubated at 36°C for three hours, or for five hours if *Pseudomonas* sp. is being tested. During this time, the cuvette is shaken to insure proper suspension of the organism and rapid elution of the antimicrobic from the discs. After three to five hours of incubation, the cuvette is removed and placed on the carriage of the photometer, where the amount of light scattered by each chamber is measured automatically.

LIGHT-SCATTERING MEASUREMENT PRINCIPLE

The principle of the measurement of forward light scattering is portrayed in Figure 10-4. The cuvette's optical chamber is shown in

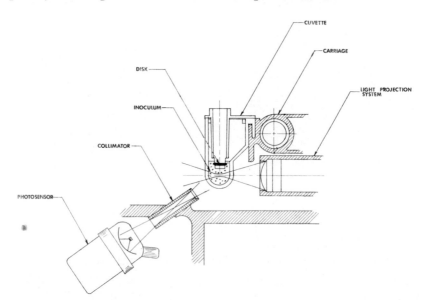

Figure 10-4. Optical arrangement of cuvette in photometer, showing location of elution disc and inoculated broth.

cross section. The amount of light scattered at a 35° angle is measured by the photodetector through the collimating tube. The value obtained is directly proportional to the number of microorganisms and may be used as a sensitive index of the bacterial population.

For reading, the cuvette is placed in the Autobac I photometer, the door closed, and the reporting ticket inserted. The photometer then automatically reads the light-scattering value in each chamber and calculates a light-scattering index (LSI) for each antimicrobic. From this light-scattering index, the photometer assigns a susceptible, equivocal, or resistant interpretation to each antimicrobic tested.

The machine automatically measures the amount of light scattered by the inoculated chamber at time zero (when the inoculum is first adjusted), and this value is retained in the machine's memory and entered as a constant in future calculations.

Growth Index. The growth index is the logarithm of the ratio of the light scattered in the control chamber at the end of three hours to the light scattered at the time 0. The latter is equal to the initial inoculum standardized by the same photometer and is therefore a constant retained in the machine's memory. The growth index is a measure of the uninhibited growth of the microorganism in the absence of antimicrobic. The photometer is automatically programed to reject a cuvette if the growth index is less than 0.9, e.g., if the antilog of 0.9 equals 8, or 3 doublings of the bacterial population. In such a case, the cuvette may be returned to the incubator/shaker for an additional incubation period since the test is nondestructive.

LSI Values. A light-scattering index (LSI) is computed for each antimicrobic chamber by first calculating a growth index for each chamber with antimicrobics. This value is divided by the growth index for the control chamber. The LSI may then be defined as follows:

$$\text{LSI} = \frac{\text{Log growth index in test chamber}}{\text{Log growth index in control chamber}}$$

This formula provides an index of growth inhibition ranging from 0 to 1, an LSI of 0 representing complete resistance and an LSI of 1 representing complete susceptibility. These LSI values are then interpreted by the instrument as resistance, equivocal, or susceptible according to criteria that have been defined to correlate with the interpretation of disc diffusion tests. An LSI of 0 to 0.50 is resistant, 0.51-0.59 is equivocal, and 0.60-1 is susceptible with all antimicrobics except penicillin, in which case an LSI of 0 to 0.90 is resistant and an LSI of 0.91 to 1 is susceptible. Interpretation of results of tests with penicillin G must be noted manually on the report form.

LIMITATIONS

When ampicillin and cephalothin are being tested, some *Enterobacter* sp. produce small clumps of bacteria that may not be detected by the scanning beam but can be seen on the bottom of the cuvette when manually examined. Thus they may appear susceptible in the three-hour Autobac system but resistant by the overnight disc diffusion test. Barry and colleagues[1] have demonstrated that disc diffusion tests may be read as early as four to five hours after inoculation. Small, clear zones of inhibition were often seen with *Enterobacter* sp. tested against ampicillin or cephalothin or with *Serratia* sp. tested against the polymyxins; after overnight incubation, nearly confluent colonies were seen growing within these initially clear zones. In the light of that observation, it is not surprising that the early rapid tests with the Autobac system might occasionally indicate susceptibility and the standard tests indicate resistance. Major discrepancies might also occur with *Pseudomonas aeruginosa* or enterococci tested against tetracycline or with *Staphylococcus epidermidis* tested against methicillin or penicillin G. Because of the inducible nature of staphylococcal penicillin β-lactamase (Chapter 9), a minimal inhibition of growth (LSI 0.90 or less) is considered evidence of resistance, and a LSI of 0.91 or greater is required before the strain may be considered susceptible. With this modification, the Autobac system appears to provide a reliable distinction between penicillin-susceptible and penicillin-resistant strains of *S. aureus*. Its ability to detect methicillin-resistant strains of *S. aureus* has not yet been documented.

The Autobac system cannot be used to test enterococci with cephalothin, streptomycin, neomycin, or doxycycline nor to test pseudomonads against kanamycin or streptomycin nor to test *S. epidermidis* against ampicillin, and therefore tests with these combinations are contraindicated. This is not a major disadvantage to the test system since these particular combinations of drugs and microorganisms are not especially relevant clinically.

Since the Autobac system employs a broth method, it is not possible to determine when readings are being taken on mixed cultures. Because mixed cultures can be extremely unreliable, every precaution must be exercised to insure pure cultures in the initial inoculum. After standardization of each saline suspension, a drop or loopful should be transferred to a suitable nutrient agar plate and streaked for isolation. These "purity checks" should be examined after overnight incubation; if a mixed culture is found, the tests should be repeated and a corrective report issued.

As with most other susceptibility tests, the Autobac system is unable to test nutritionally fastidious pathogens or obligate anaerobes or capnophiles. However, it should be possible to modify the medium or the cuvette in order to permit testing of such microorganisms.

For testing the common rapid-growing bacterial pathogens, this testing system has been evaluated extensively and found to give results nearly comparable to the standardized disc diffusion technique. The qualitative interpretation of results with both the automated disc elution technique and the disc diffusion methods corresponds favorably with MICs obtained with a standard agar dilution technique. In a recent collaborative study,[4] overall agreement with agar dilution MICs was approximately 90% for either method and reproducibility of results with the Autobac I and with the disc diffusion methods was equivalent.

Although this test system has not yet withstood the all-important test of time, it is one of the few semi-automated for rapid susceptibility testing that have been extensively evaluated and are now available.

REFERENCES

1. Barry, A. L., L. J. Joyce, A. P. Adams, and E. J. Benner. 1973. Rapid determination of antimicrobial susceptibility for urgent clinical situations. Am. J. Clin. Pathol. *59:* 693-699.
2. McKie, J. E., R. J. Borovoy, J. F. Dooley, G. R. Evanega, G. Mendoza, F. Meyer, M. Moody, D. E. Packer, J. Praglin, and H. Smith. 1975. Autobac 1—a 3-hour, automated antimicrobial susceptibility system. II. Microbiological studies. In *Automation in Microbiology and Immunology.* C. G. Heden and T. Illeni (Eds.). Wiley, New York. pp. 211-242.
3. Paglin, J., A. C. Curtiss, D. K. Longhenry, and J. E. McKie. 1975. Autobac 1—a 3-hour, automated antimicrobial susceptibility system I. System description. In *Automation in Microbiology and Immunology.* C. G. Heden and T. Illeni (Eds.). Wiley, New York. pp. 199-208.
4. Thornsberry, C., T. L. Gavan, J. C. Sherris, A. Balows, J. M. Matsen, L. D. Sabath, F. Schoenknecht, L. D. Thrupp, and J. A. Washington II. 1975. Laboratory evaluation of a rapid, automated susceptibility testing system: Report of a collaborative study. Antimicrob. Agents Chemother. *7:* 466-480.

Chapter **11**

ANTIMICROBIC SUSCEPTIBILITY OF YEASTS

Michael A. Saubolle

Systemic infections caused by yeasts pose major diagnostic and therapeutic problems. Until recently, the only antimycotic agents available were the polyene antimicrobics: amphotericin B, nystatin, and candicidin. Only amphotericin B could be administered parenterally and was thus the only antimycotic agent available for treating general infections. However, its use was limited by its toxicity. In the last few years, several new agents were discovered and are being evaluated or have been shown to be efficacious for treating systemic mycotic infections. To the stimulus of such developments must be added the fact of a particularly poor prognosis in patients with compromised host defenses who do not receive specific, effective therapy. The net result is to render susceptibility testing of yeasts increasingly important, if not imperative.

In principle, methods for testing the *in vitro* susceptibility of yeast are the same as those described for testing bacterial pathogens. However, susceptibility testing is somewhat more difficult because of unique biological and physicochemical properties of the yeasts and the antimycotic agents being tested.

142

ANTIMYCOTIC AGENTS AND THEIR PROPERTIES

Three antimycotic agents are presently available commercially for treating the deep-seated or systemic yeast infections: amphotericin B (AMB), nystatin (NYS), and 5-fluorocytosine (5-FC). Nystatin is too toxic for parenteral administration and is not absorbed well enough from the gastrointestinal tract to be systemically effective after oral administration. Its use is therefore limited to topical application and perhaps for mycotic gastroenteritis. AMB is not absorbed well from the gastrointestinal tract, but it can be administered parenterally in limited doses.

Both NYS and AMB are insoluble in water, unstable in acid, and inactivated by light. The activity of AMB may decline rapidly in the presence of cysteine. Thus, the test medium should be free of cysteine and the pH should approach physiologic values.

5-FC is soluble in water, well absorbed from the gastrointestinal tract, stable, and relatively nontoxic. It is fungistatic rather than fungicidal, depending on metabolic conversion to 5-fluorouracil in the yeast cell for antifungal activity. For susceptibility testing with 5-FC, it is essential to use a culture medium that does not contain either cytosine or uridine. Although yeasts are often susceptible to 5-FC on primary isolation, resistance may develop during treatment.

A fourth antimycotic agent, clotrimazole (CLO), is an imidazole derivative that has been studied extensively in Europe. Although very active *in vitro*, it is so poorly tolerated on oral administration that it cannot be used clinically. However, it is effective on topical application for treating superficial mycoses.

Newer antimycotic agents not yet available for general use include amphotericin B methyl ester and miconazole. Preliminary experiments with these agents have been promising.

Amphotericin B methyl ester (AME) was prepared at Rutgers University by molecular alteration of AMB. Its advantages over AMB include solubility in aqueous systems at physiologic pH and diminished toxicity. However, AME, like AMB, is sensitive to light and acid, and thus one must apply the precautions used in testing with AMB to testing with AME. Furthermore, AME is readily oxidized once dissolved in water, and thus storage of stock solutions is not advised.

Miconazole (MCZ) is an investigational imidazole derivative that may be useful in systemic and topical antifungal therapy. Miconazole is virtually insoluble in water, but it can be administered intravenously as a colloidal suspension stabilized with polyethoxylated castor oil. Preliminary results have been promising and serious adverse reactions from its use have been negligible.

Preparation and Storage of Stock Solutions. For susceptibility testing of yeasts, stock solutions of most antimycotic agents can be prepared and stored under the proper conditions until needed for further dilution.

AMB and NYS are available in two forms. As standard powders (Squibb) they can be dissolved in either dimethylsulfoxide (DMSO) or in dimethylformamide to give concentrations of 5,000 μg/ml. These solutions should be allowed to autosterilize for about 30 minutes in the dark before use. AMB is also available as Fungizone (Squibb), a sterile powder suitable for intravenous injection after suspension in 5% glucose solution. Nystatin is available as a colloidal suspension for use in tissue culture media (Grand Island Biological Co.). Both of these polyene suspensions can be diluted in sterile distilled water to give the required concentration and can be stored frozen in the dark for at least one week.

5-FC, available as a white standard powder (Hoffmann-LaRoche), can be dissolved in distilled water to make a 10,000 μg/ml stock solution. Sterilized by filtration, the solution can be stored almost indefinitely at $-30°$C.

CLO is available as a standard powder (BAY-5097, Delbay Pharmaceuticals) for research testing. It is insoluble in water but can be dissolved in organic solvents, such as 95% ethanol or DMSO. A stock solution of 3448 μg/ml (10 μ moles/ml) in ethanol can be filter sterilized and stored almost indefinitely at $-30°$C in the dark. Further dilutions can be made with sterile distilled water when needed. With the addition of water, a precipitate may appear, but it does not alter the activity of CLO in susceptibility tests.

At present, AME, is available only as a powder for research purposes. It can be dissolved in distilled water to give the required stock solutions and sterilized by filtration. Because it is even less stable in solution than either NYS or AMB, AME should be kept in the dark and used as soon as possible after the solutions are prepared.

MCZ is available as a sterile aqueous suspension suitable for intravenous injection (Janssen Pharmaceutica, Belgium). The concentration is 8,700 μg/ml, and the drug is stable almost indefinitely at 4°C. Dilutions should be made with sterile distilled water.

GENERAL CONSIDERATIONS

Different investigators have advocated different techniques for testing the susceptibility of yeasts *in vitro*. Several of these

methods have been used quite regularly, apparently with good correlation with the clinical outcome of the therapeutic regimen. As
with bacterial susceptibility testing, results obtained in the testing
of yeasts are related to the inoculum size, time of incubation, incubation temperature, and medium used. Because these parameters
are not yet standardized, results from different laboratories are
often in disagreement. Standardization within a given laboratory is
essential before a regular program of susceptibility testing of yeasts
can be instituted.

A single standard method is difficult to define because different
methods may have to be employed for testing different agents and
different yeasts (e.g., *Candida*, *Torulopsis*, and *Cryptococcus*). For
example, yeast nitrogen base (YNB, Difco) is preferred by some
workers for tests with 5-FC, and antibiotic medium 20 (M-20, Difco) is commonly used for testing AMB, NYS, and AME.

Of all the methods for *in vitro* susceptibility testing of yeasts, the
broth dilution technique is probably the best suited for general
application in the microbiology laboratory. The agar dilution
method has shown good correlation with the broth dilution method,
and it may be used when large numbers of isolates are to be tested
at one time. Disc agar diffusion techniques have shown much
promise but have not yet been sufficiently standardized to be
applicable to clinical work. Research is now in progress, and a
better standardized test method may be forthcoming in the near
future. Finally, the microdilution technique may also be applied to
susceptibility testing of yeasts. This method, however, has not been
used as often as the macrodilution technique, and more experience
is needed before it can be implemented on a regular basis.

Choice of Medium. The choice of medium depends on the antifungal agent being tested. With some agents, activity may be obfus-
cated by the medium.

For testing with 5-FC, yeast nitrogen base (YNB, Difco),
supplemented with glucose and asparagine,[11] is often recommended. It can be stored at 4°C as a 10 × concentrate, ready to be
diluted 1:10 with sterile distilled water as needed. However, YNB
is too acidic (pH 5.5) for testing AMB, AME, NYS, CLO, or MCZ,
and it is essentially unbuffered. The polyenes CLO and MCZ are
often tested in antibiotic medium 20 (M-20, Difco), which has a
higher initial pH (6.6).

In an attempt to standardize a single, non-obfuscating medium
for susceptibility testing of fungi, a synthetic amino acid medium
for fungi (SAAMF) was devised by Hoeprich et al.[6] This medium
can be used for testing with all the commercially available antifun-

gal agents, as well as with the newer agents, such as AME and the imidazole derivatives.

SAAMF has a pH of 7.4. It is exceptionally well buffered by means of a synthetic, nonchelating, weak acid–weak base pair, and contains neither macromolecules nor purines or pyrimidines. The formula for the preparation of SAAMF is given in Table 11-1. It can be prepared as a 2 × concentrate, stored at 4°C for several weeks, and diluted with sterile, distilled water as needed.

Table 11-1. Synthetic Amino Acid Medium, Fungal (SAAMF)

Ingredients and method of preparation of 1-liter

Solution I (1-liter flask):

MEM Amino Acids (TC Amino Acids Minimal Eagle, Dried [Difco Laboratories, Detroit])

Use 10-liter size (Code 5856), i.e., 5.09 gm:

l-Arginine	1.05 gm	*l*-Cystine	0.24 gm
l-Lysine	0.58 gm	*l*-Methionine	0.15 gm
l-Histidine	0.31 gm		
		l-Threonine	0.48 gm
l-Tyrosine	0.36 gm	*l*-Leucine	0.52 gm
l-Tryptophane	0.10 gm	*l*-Isoleucine	0.52 gm
l-Phenylalanine	0.32 gm	*l*-Valine	0.46 gm

Dissolve in 350 ml distilled water, heating gently (37°-40°C) with constant stirring for 15 to 20 minutes. Set flask aside and allow insoluble components (possibly, cystine and tyrosine) to settle out. Meanwhile, prepare Solution II.

Solution II:

Weigh into a 2-liter flask:

d-Glucose	20.0 gm	*l*-Glutamine	2.52 gm
Fumaric acid	1.50 gm	*l*-Asparagine	1.00 gm
Na pyruvate	1.00 gm	*l*-Proline	1.00 gm
NH_4 acetate	0.25 gm	Glycine	0.50 gm
$K_2HPO_4 \cdot 3H_2O$	0.50 gm	MOPS[1]	16.45 gm
		Tris[2]	10.45 gm

Decant supernatant Solution I into flask containing ingredients of Solution II.

Dissolve residue of Solution I in 0.3 ml 10 N NaOH. Add to Solution II, washing flash twice with 2 or 3 ml distilled water.

Heat Solution II gently (37°-40°C), with constant stirring. Add, in order: 0.2% phenol red—1 ml; mineral solution[3]—1 ml; and 50 ml BME vitamins.[4] Set pH to 7.4 (10 N NaOH) and add sufficient distilled water to make final volume to 500 ml.

Sterilize by membrane filtration.

The above is 2 X concentration: To use as SAAMF liquid medium, mix with an equal volume of sterile distilled water.

For SAAMF agar, suspend 10 gm Ionagar No. 2S (Wilson Diagnostics, Inc., 3 Science Road, Glenwood, Ill. 60425) in 500 ml distilled water. Autoclave. Cool to 45°C and add to 500 ml of liquid 2 X SAAMF previously warmed to 45°C.

STANDARDIZATION OF INOCULUM DENSITY

As in susceptibility testing with bacteria, the inoculum size is a critical factor in testing the susceptibility of yeasts. A standardized cell suspension can be obtained by one of two methods:

1. The yeast is incubated for 24 to 48 hours in 5 ml of the appropriate broth medium at 36° to 37°C (Sabouraud's broth should not be used for growing isolates to be tested with 5-FC, CLO, or MCZ because of the possibility of antagonism). The number of organisms per ml can be ascertained by direct counting in a hemacytometer.

Alternatively, 24-to-48-hour broth cultures can be assumed to contain approximately 10^7 to 10^8 colony-forming units (CFU) per ml. Some yeasts, such as *Cryptococcus* sp., may require longer incubation periods to approach a stationary phase. When different species of yeasts are being tested, this approach is least practical because of marked differences in the time required to reach the maximal cell concentration, even under similar test conditions. Furthermore, some yeasts (especially *Candida* sp.) produce mycelial elements and clumping in the broth medium. Thus, blind dilution of 24-to-48-hour broth cultures is recommended only for reference strains that have been found by previous experimentation to give predictable results (that is, when a few standard strains are being used for experimental studies).

2. Discrete colonies selected from a one-to-two-day-old agar plate can be suspended in 2 to 4 ml of 0.9% NaCl solution and then adjusted to give an optical density of 0.5 absorbance at 540 nm (Bausch & Lomb Spectronic 20 Colorimeter). Such a suspension contains about 10^7 CFU/ml, but the exact number varies somewhat with different colorimeters and with different yeasts. The use of optical density for the preparation of a standard suspension is likely to be reproducible if considera-

---

[1] MOPS = 2-(N-morpholino) propane sulfonic acid

[2] Tris = 2-amino-2-(hydroxymethyl)-1,3-propanediol

[3] Mineral solution:

Solution A:		Solution B (the working solution):	
$FeCl_3 \cdot 6H_2O$	6.75 gm	$CaCl_2 \cdot 6H_2O$	1.10 gm
$ZnSO_4 \cdot 7H_2O$	2.00 gm	$MgCl_2 \cdot 6H_2O$	20.33 gm
$MnSO_4 \cdot 4H_2O$	0.90 gm	Conc. HCl	0.5 ml
Conc. HCl	12.5 ml	Solution A	1.0 ml
Distilled water *q.s. ad*	25.0 ml	Distilled water *q.s. ad*	100 ml

[4] Vitamins (BME Vitamin Solution [100X] [Grand Island Biological Company, 2323 Fifth Street, Berkeley, Calif. 94710])

Vitamin	mg/l	Vitamin	mg/l
Biotin	100	Pyridoxal HCl	100
Folic acid	100	Thiamine HCl	100
Choline chloride	100	Riboflavin	10
Nicotinamide	100	i-Inositol	180
d-Ca pentothenate	100		

NOTE: For testing bacteria, the same medium (SAAM) may be prepared with 0.025 gm uracil per l and with only 0.5 gm glucose per l. (From P. D. Hoeprich and A. C. Huston. 1975. Susceptibility of *Coccidioides immitis, Candida albicans,* and *Cryptococcus neoformans* to amphotericin B, flucytosine, and clotrimazole. J. Infect. Dis., *132:*133-141.)

tion is given to the calibration of the colorimeter and the yeast species being tested (e.g., to the fact that at a given optical density the number of cells of a *Torulopsis* sp. will be slightly greater than the number of *Candida* sp.). The suspensions should be thoroughly mixed to minimize the effect of clumping.

BROTH DILUTION TECHNIQUE

The broth dilution technique is probably the most widely used method for susceptibility testing of yeasts. It is also the simplest and most practical method presently available for testing individual isolates. It not only provides the MIC of an antifungal agent but also can be extended to provide information concerning the lethal activity (MIC) of the agent. Dilutions of antimicrobics can be prepared ahead of time and stored frozen until needed (with the exception of AME).

The broth dilution technique can be utilized with only a few basic changes in procedure for the susceptibility testing of all yeast species. The medium, inoculum size, temperature of incubation, and time of reading the results are major parameters that need to be standardized. Any deviation from the procedure chosen may drastically change the results of the test. The actual procedures depend on the antimicrobic and the yeast being tested.

Serial Dilution of Antifungal Agents. The procedure for making the dilutions of each antifungal agent is the same for all yeasts and agents being tested. The series of dilutions for each agent must extend above and below the attainable serum levels of that agent. A suggested series for each drug, with its approximate maximum serum level, is shown in Table 11-2 (this can be adjusted to the specific needs of the individual laboratory).

The dilutions can be prepared in advance at $10 \times$ concentration, dispensed in 0.1-ml amounts into 12-by-75-mm disposable plastic tubes, tightly capped, and stored frozen at $-20°C$ until required. Storage beyond two weeks is not recommended without appropriate controls; tubes with AME should be used immediately. In every case, once a tube is thawed for use it should be discarded if not used the same day. The series of tubes needed for testing should be thawed as close as possible to the time of use to insure full potency.

Preparation of Inoculum. The specific size of the inoculum still remains somewhat arbitrary; the literature contains reports of tests performed with inocula as low as 10^2 and as high as 10^6 organisms per ml, with rather drastic differences in results. An attempt to reproduce test conditions resembling the *in vivo* environment probably favors a fairly large inoculum. Although there are no quantitative assessments of the actual concentration of yeast cells

Table 11-2. Suggested Dilution Schedule for Antimycotic Agents to be Tested by Broth Dilution and Agar Dilution Susceptibility Techniques

Tube #	Amphotericin B MW: 960.34		Amphotericin B Methylester MW: 974.37		5-Fluorocytosine MW: 129.1		Clotrimazole MW: 344.8		Miconazole MW: 479.16	
	10 ×* Conc. (μg/ml)	Final Conc. (μg/ml)	10 ×* Conc. (μg/ml)	Final Conc. (μg/ml)	10 ×* Conc. (μg/ml)	Final Conc. (μg/ml)	10 ×* Conc. (μg/ml)	Final Conc. (μg/ml)	10 ×* Conc. (μg/ml)	Final Conc. (μg/ml)
1	100.0	10.0	200.0	20.0	3200.0	320.0	150.0	15.0	200.0	20.0
2	50.0	5.0	100.0	10.0	1600.0	160.0	75.0	7.5	100.0	10.0
3	25.0	2.5†	50.0	5.0	800.0	80.0†	37.5	3.75	50.0	5.0†
4	12.5	1.25	25.0	2.5	400.0	40.0	18.75	1.875†	25.0	2.5
5	6.25	0.625	12.5	1.25	200.0	20.0	9.375	0.9375	12.5	1.25
6	3.125	0.3125	6.25	0.625	100.0	10.0	4.6875	0.4688	6.25	0.625
7	1.5625	0.15625	3.125	0.3125	50.0	5.0	2.3438	0.2344	3.125	0.3125

* 0.1 ml of the 10 × concentration of antimycotic agent is distributed to each appropriate tube. On the test day 0.9 ml of inoculum broth is added to these tubes, resulting in the final 1 × concentration. For agar dilution tests, a 1:10 dilution of the drug is accomplished by adding 2 ml of stock solution to 18 ml of agar medium.

† Approximate highest attainable serum levels.

involved in different infections, a realistic value might easily approach 10^4 or 10^5 ml. However, when testing *Cryptococcus* sp., Bennett[3] found the most reproducible results by using an inoculum density of 10^2 organisms per ml. At the present time, the best choice for inoculum size is: (1) approximately 10^4 organisms per ml when testing the genera *Candida, Torulopsis, Rhodotorula, Saccharomyces*, and *Trichosporon* and (2) approximately 10^2 organisms per ml when testing the genus *Cryptococcus*.

Inocula are obtained by diluting the standardized cell suspension described above. Preparation of the standardized suspensions and inocula should be done just prior to the time of the susceptibility tests.

Broth Dilution Susceptibility Testing Procedure. With the series of drug concentrations prepared in advance and stored frozen, the standardized cell suspensions can be prepared while the tubes of drugs are thawing and warming to room temperature. The final dilution of the inoculum is carried out in the appropriate test broth medium to provide approximately 10^4 organisms per ml. The diluted, final inoculum suspension is then distributed in 0.9-ml volumes to each of the test tubes in each drug series, including control tubes without antimicrobics. The addition of 0.9 ml of the yeast cell suspension to the 0.1 ml of 10 × concentration of test drug dilutes the latter to the desired concentration but does not significantly dilute the yeast inoculum.

In addition to the test yeast strain, a control strain of known susceptibility should be tested with each drug series to document the potency of the drug. Strains previously tested or strains selected from the American Type Culture Collection (e.g., *Saccharomyces cerevisiae* ATCC 9763, *S. cerevisiae* ATCC 2601, or *Candida tropicalis* ATCC 13803) are suitable for use as controls. In addition, each series of drug dilutions should include: (1) two growth control tubes with no drug (one incubated with the tests, the other refrigerated until the tests are read) and (2) a tube containing 0.1 ml of the highest final drug concentration plus 0.9 ml of un-inoculated broth (sterility control).

Incubation and Reading. The MIC results can be read after either 24 or 48 hours of incubation at 35°C, depending on the drugs and yeast strains being tested. Isolates of *Cryptococcus* sp. usually replicate slowly, and incubation periods must be extended to at least 48 hours. With 5-FC, tests should always be read after 48 hours to detect the delayed growth of resistant variants. When testing the polyenes, results should be read as soon as possible because of drug instability at the higher temperature. Unfortunately, 24-hour readings may not be possible with some *Cryptococcus* sp. and with some *Candida* sp. Accordingly, tests should be examined daily until growth appears in the drug-free control tubes, at which time the MIC is determined.

The MIC is defined as the lowest concentration of antifungal agent that inhibits visible growth of the yeast. All tubes should be thoroughly mixed and then examined by transmitted light. The MLC can be determined by subculturing 0.05 ml (5% of the volume) from each tube without visible growth and from the growth control tube onto either Sabouraud's glucose agar or brain-heart infusion agar. The MLC is the lowest concentration of drug from which subculturing yields five or fewer colonies (99.9% kill). Normally, the MLCs can be read after 24 to 48 hours of incubation at 35°C, i.e., when growth is apparent on the control plate.

End-points with the polyenes are normally clear-cut, but with 5-FC and with the imidazole derivatives, a progressive decline in the amount of growth is often seen with each increase in drug concentration. Often the growth is so scant that difficulty is encountered in discriminating between actual growth and a slight haziness found in the test medium. As in bacterial susceptibility testing, the presence of a very light haziness is regarded as negative. To help define the MIC end-points, the tests should be compared against two control tubes: (1) the un-inoculated sterility control incubated with the test series of tubes and (2) an inoculated tube kept at 4° to 8°C to inhibit growth. Such control tubes help in distinguishing actual growth from precipitated drug or inoculum in the test medium.

AGAR DILUTION TECHNIQUE

The agar dilution technique is a simple method for the susceptibility testing of yeasts that is especially useful when a large number of isolates are to be tested at one time. Many of the principles outlined for broth dilution are also applicable to the agar dilution technique.

Selection of Medium and Preparation of Plates. The principles governing the selection of a test medium are the same as those used in the choice of medium for the broth dilution technique; the choice depends on the antifungal agent against which the yeast is being tested. The synthetic broth medium can be prepared in a 2 × concentration and refrigerated until needed. For testing, agar (Ionagar No. 2, Wilson Diagnostics, Inc.) is dissolved in distilled water to give a 2% solution (2 × concentration), autoclaved, and placed in a 50°C water bath to cool. At the same time, an equal volume of 2 × test medium should be warmed to 50°C in the water bath. Mixing equal volumes provides the required concentration of test medium in 1% molten agar. The appropriate amount of medium (18 ml for preparation of 15-by-100-mm petri plates) is then dispensed into sterile, screw-cap tubes.

Serial Dilution of Antimycotic Agents. The drug dilutions should be prepared in 10 × concentrations of the final values required for the agar test plates (Table 11-2). The dilutions should be prepared from the stock solutions as close as possible to the time of use to minimize possible inactivation of the drugs (e.g., AMB, AME). Once the drug dilutions are ready and 18 ml of the melted agar medium has been dispensed to glass tubes, 2 ml of each 10 × drug concentrate is added to the agar medium, immediately mixed by inversion, and poured into a 15-by-100-mm plastic petri dish. The plates, which should have been appropriately labeled prior to pouring, are ready for use immediately after gelling. They should not be stored.

Inoculum. A standardized inoculum is prepared as for the broth dilution technique. A 1:2 dilution of a suspension containing 10^7 organisms per ml provides an inoculum size of about 5×10^6 organisms per ml. When the inoculum is applied with an inoculator that transfers 0.001 to 0.003 ml, about 10^3 to 10^4 organisms are deposited per total spot inoculation. If other devices are used to spot-inoculate the plates, the volume transferred must be determined so that appropriate dilutions of the stock suspension can be made.

Agar Dilution Procedure. While the serial drug plates are being prepared, the inoculum is standardized and diluted. The plates are spot-inoculated, using a sterile replicator as described for tests with bacteria. The plates are then placed in the incubator with their lids partially open to allow the inocula to dry (to avoid possible running of the inocula). When excess fluid has evaporated (30 minutes to one hour), the lids are replaced and the plates are inverted for incubation at 35°C.

Tests should be read as soon as the control plate becomes positive, except that with 5-FC a final determination is not made before 48 hours. The MIC is defined as the lowest concentration of drug that inhibits growth on the plate; inoculated spots having three or more colonies are considered positive. The inoculated microorganisms often undergo several replications before being inhibited by the drug, producing a hazy film in the inoculated area. Such a film of growth should be considered negative.

Table 11-3. Expected Ranges of SAAMF Broth Dilution MIC and MLC Values (μg/ml) of Five Antimycotic Agents against Five Yeast Species Implicated in Systemic Infection

Yeast	Amphotericin B		Amphotericin B Methyl Ester		5-Fluorocytosine		Clotrimazole		Miconazole	
	MIC	MLC	MIC	MLC	MIC	MLC	MIC	MLC	MIC	MLC
Candida * *albicans*	≤0.6	≤0.6 - 1.2 (≤0.6)‡	≤0.6 - 2.4 (0.8)	1.2 - >9.7 (1.2)	≤10 - >322 (≤10)	≤10 - >322 (>322)	≤0.22 - >6.9 (≤0.22)	1.7 - >6.9 (>6.9)	≤0.6 - >19 (≤0.6)	>19
Candida * *tropicalis*	≤0.6	≤0.6	≤0.6 - 1.2 (1.2)	1.2 - 2.4 (1.2)	≤10 - >322 (≤10)	20 - >322 (20)	≤0.22	≤0.22 - 0.86 (≤0.22)	≤0.6 - 1.2 (≤0.6)	0.6 >19 (0.9)
Candida * *parapsilosis*	≤0.6	≤0.6 - >4.8 (≤0.6)	≤0.6 - 2.4 (2.4)	1.2 - 4.8 (2.4)	≤10 - 40 (≤10)	40 - >322 (>322)	≤0.22 - 0.86 (≤0.22)	≤0.22 - >6.9 (>6.9)	≤0.6 - >19 (≤0.6)	9.6 - >19 (>19)
Torulopsis * *glabrata*	≤0.6	≤0.6 - 2.4 (≤0.6)	≤0.6 - 2.4 (1.2)	≤0.6 - 4.8 (2.0)	≤10 - >322 (≤10)	≤10 - >322 (≤10)	0.86 - >6.9 (1.72)	>6.9	≤0.6 - 2.4 (≤0.6)	>19
Cryptococcus† *neoformans*	≤0.6 - 4.8 (≤0.6)	≤0.6 - 4.8 (≤0.6)	≤0.6 - 4.8 (2.4)	≤0.8 - 4.8 (2.4)	≤10 - >322 (≤10)	≤10 - >322 (>322)	≤0.22 - >6.9 (≤0.22)	≤0.22 - >6.9 (3.45)	≤0.6	≤0.6 - >19 (4.79)

SOURCE: Saubolle and Hoeprich. Unpublished data.

NOTE: No. of isolates tested: *C. albicans* = 84; *C. tropicalis* = 6; *C. parapsilosis* = 8; *T. glabrata* = 22; *C. neoformans* = 7.

* MIC readings taken at 24 hours; MLC subcultures taken at 48 hours.

† MIC readings taken at 48 hours.

‡ Mode.

SUSCEPTIBILITY TESTING OF YEASTS: OVERVIEW

The need for standardization, elucidation of significance, and acceptance of yeast susceptibility tests has become pressing as the numbers of yeast infections and of antimycotic agents increase. Currently, there is considerable disagreement as to the appropriate methods of testing, the significance of results, and even the need for testing with some antifungals. Communication between laboratories and standardization of methods would clear up many of the disagreements; once results can be compared, their significance to the clinical situation might become better appreciated.

Even at present, however, yeast susceptibility tests can provide valuable information on the possible efficacy of a drug or the emergence of drug resistance during therapy of a yeast infection. Although interpretation of results is often difficult, a range of MICs reported for several yeasts is listed in Table 11-3. On the whole, both the treatment of fungal infections and susceptibility testing of the organisms involved are more difficult than the treatment and susceptibility testing of the better-known bacterial counterparts.

REFERENCES

1. Bennett, J. E. 1974. Chemotherapy of systemic mycoses. I. N. Engl. J. Med. *290:* 30-32.
2. Bennett, J. E. 1974. Chemotherapy of systemic mycoses. II. N. Engl. J. Med. *290:* 320-323.
3. Block, E. R., A. E. Jennings, and J. E. Bennett. 1973. Variables influencing susceptibility testing of *Cryptococcus neoformans* to 5-fluorocytosine. Antimicrob. Agents Chemother. *4:* 392-395.
4. Burgess, M. A., and G. P. Bodey. 1972. Clotrimazole (Bay b 5097): *In vitro* and clinical pharmacological studies. Antimicrob. Agents Chemother. *2:* 423-426.
5. Hamilton-Miller, J. M. T. 1972. A comparative *in vitro* study of amphotericin B, clotrimazole and 5-fluorocytosine against clinically isolated yeasts. Sabouraudia *10:* 276-283.
6. Hoeprich, P. D., and P. D. Finn. 1972. Obfuscation of the activity of antifungal antimicrobics by culture media. J. Infect. Dis. *126:* 353-361.
7. Hoeprich, P. D., and A. C. Huston. 1975. Susceptibility of *Coccidioides immitis, Candida albicans* and *Cryptococcus neoformans* to amphotericin B, flucytosine, and clotrimzole. J. Infect. Dis., *132:* 133-141.
8. Holt, R. J. 1974. Recent developments in antimycotic chemotherapy. Infection *2:* 95-107.
9. Marks, M. I., and T. C. Eickhoff. 1970. Application of four methods to the study of the susceptibility of yeast to 5-fluorocytosine. Antimicrob. Agents Chemother. *10:* 491-493.
10. Shadomy, S., and A. E. Ingroff. 1974. Susceptibility testing of antifungal agents. In: *The Manual of Clinical Microbiology*, 2d ed. E. H. Lennette, E. H. Spaulding, and J. P. Traunt (Eds.). American Society for Microbiology, Washington, D. C. pp. 569-574.
11. Shadomy, S., C. B. Kirchoff, and A. E. Ingroff. 1973. *In vitro* activity of 5-fluorocytosine against *Candida* and *Torulopsis* species. Antimicrob. Agents Chemother. *3:* 9-14.

Chapter 12

ANTIMICROBIC SUSCEPTIBILITY OF *MYCOBACTERIUM* SP.

Once the diagnosis of tuberculosis has been established, chemotherapy may be initiated with at least two of the so-called primary drugs, namely, isoniazid (INH), ethambutol, streptomycin, rifampin, and *p*-aminosalicyclic acid (PAS). The reason for using a combination of two or more drugs is related to the fact that many strains of *M. tuberculosis* contain a fairly small proportion of resistant variants among an otherwise fully susceptible population. Therapy with a single drug may select the resistant portion of the population, eventually resulting in a therapeutic failure. However, when a second, unrelated, drug is also administered, the resistant variants that are not inhibited by the first drug are eliminated by the second one. For that reason, antimicrobic susceptibility tests of *Mycobacterium* sp. must be capable of detecting a relatively low proportion of resistant cells within each population. Extensive experience has shown that when more than 1% of a bacillary population has become resistant to one of the primary drugs, it does not continue to be useful, i.e., the 1% soon becomes the predominant form if therapy with that drug alone is continued. Cell populations containing less than 1% resistant forms are generally considered susceptible to that drug. The proportion of resistant variants within a population can best be detected by an agar dilution type of procedure. The susceptibility of *Mycobacterium* sp. is usually tested by inoculating the surface of an agar medium containing a fixed concentration of the antimicrobic in question and determining the number of resistant cells within the inoculum.

In patients who have never been treated previously, the pathogen is likely to be susceptible to the primary drugs and therapy is usually initiated as soon as the diagnosis is established, pending the results of susceptibility tests. There is a greater probability that drug-resistant organisms have emerged in patients who have been treated previously with anti-tuberculosis drugs, or when adequately controlled therapy has failed to convert the patient to a negative-culture status within a few months. Because drug resistance is commonly seen among retreatment patients, it might be appropriate to withhold therapy from them until susceptibility tests can be performed. In such cases, drug-susceptibility tests must be carried out as quickly as possible.

To minimize the delay before the susceptibility test results are reported, drug-susceptibility plates may be inoculated directly with the concentrated clinical specimen, provided that it contains a sufficiently dense inoculum, i.e., if direct microscopic examination of the material reveals acid-fast bacilli. In fact, the direct procedure provides a better estimate of the proportion of drug-susceptible and drug-resistant bacilli within the specimen. With this approach it is essential that one include sufficient controls to be sure that the inoculum density is neither too light nor too heavy.

In situations in which the direct susceptibility test cannot be carried out, an indirect drug-susceptibility test may be performed using a subculture from the primary culture as the inoculum. Such a delayed test is necessary when: (1) the original specimen is smear negative but culture positive, (2) growth on the direct test is inadequate for a reliable report, or (3) one is dealing with reference cultures sent by another laboratory.

The generally accepted methods for determining drug susceptibility of *Mycobacterium* sp. are based on growth on a solid medium containing individual drugs.[2,3] In many ways the general technique involves most of the principles outlined for agar dilution tests of bacteria, except that serial dilutions of each antimicrobic are normally not incorporated into the system but, rather, only one or two concentrations of each drug are utilized. The test is somewhat more complicated by the necessarily prolonged incubation period and by technical problems involved in obtaining a satisfactorily uniform inoculum.

Agar Medium. Coagulated egg media are not particularly satis-factory since many of the drugs are heat labile and are partially inactivated during inspissation of the media. The constituents of various types of egg yolk media may bind and inactivate certain antimycobacterial drugs. Use of Middlebrook's 7H10 or 7H11 medium is generally recommended for susceptibility testing with the primary drugs. The latter medium consists of Middlebrook's 7H10 agar with pancreatic digest of casein (1 g/l). Either medium may be prepared from a 7H10 agar base and OADC (oleic acid, albumin, dextrose, and catalase) enrichment. Care must be taken not to overheat the base during sterilization.

Preparation of Stock Drug Solutions. It is possible to prepare stock solutions of each of the primary drugs as with other antimi-crobics and to store aliquots at –20°C for as long as three to six months without significant loss of activity. However, filter-paper discs containing appropriate concentrations of the primary anti-tuberculosis drugs are now commercially available and provide a convenient method for adding the drug to the agar plates. This approach avoids the need for preparing stock solutions and the possibility of error or loss of activity during storage.[1,2,4]

Preparation of Drug Media. The discs containing standardized amounts of drugs are placed in individual quadrants of divided petri dishes and 5-ml amounts of drug-free 7H10 or 7H11 agar are pipetted over the disc in each quadrant (Table 12-1). This technique not only permits preparation of just the number of plates needed for immediate use but also eliminates labeling error since the discs carry identification codes and so the drug and concentra-tion in each quadrant is apparent at a glance. The medium is then allowed to solidify and is incubated overnight in order to permit un-iform diffusion of the drug and to confirm sterility of the medium. The medium may then be used immediately or stored in sealed bags for a maximum of four weeks.

Preparation of Inoculum. For the direct method, the digested clinical specimen is diluted according to the number of acid-fast bacilli seen in the stained smear. If there is less than one acid-fast bacillus per oil immersion field, the specimen is used undiluted; if there are from one to ten acid-fast bacilli per oil immersion field, a 1:10 dilution is prepared; and if more than ten acid-fast bacilli are seen, a 1:100 dilution is used as the inoculum. Each drug-containing quadrant and one drug-free control quadrant are inocu-lated with 0.1 ml of the adjusted material. A second control quad-rant is always inoculated with the inoculum further diluted 1:100 in

Table 12-1. Distribution of Drug-Containing Discs for Susceptibility Tests of *Mycobacterium* sp.

Plate No.	Quadrant No.	Drug	Amt. (μg) Per Disk	Final Drug Conc. (μg ml)
1	I	(Control No. 1)	—	0
	II	Isoniazid	1	0.2
	III	Isoniazid	5	1.0
	IV	Ethambutol	25	5.0
2	I	(Control No. 2)	—	0
	II	Streptomycin	10	2.0
	III	Streptomycin	50	10.0
	IV	Rifampin	5	1.0
3	I	p-Aminosalicylic acid	10	2.0
	II	p-Aminosalicylic acid	50	10.0
	III	—	—	—
	IV	—	—	—

SOURCE: E. H. Runyon, A. G. Karlson, G. P. Kubica, and L. C. Wayne. 1974. In *Manual of Clinical Microbiology*, 2d ed. E. H. Lennette, E. H. Spaulding, and J. P. Truant (Eds.). American Society for Microbiology, Washington, D. C. p. 171.

order to provide a direct estimate of the number of colony-forming units actually delivered to the drug quadrants.

When the indirect method is to be used, the inoculum may be prepared from young, actively growing cultures by scraping colonies from the surface of the medium, taking care to sample all parts of the culture. The growth is suspended in about 4 ml of Dubos Tween-albumin broth containing three or four sterile glass beads. This suspension is then placed on a vortex mixer for about one minute, using precautions to obtain only swirling centrifugal mixing in order to avoid aerosol production. The suspension is then allowed to stand for 15 minutes or longer to allow the large particles to settle. The supernate is then removed and further diluted with additional Tween-albumin broth until the turbidity matches that of a No. 1 MacFarland standard. From this barely turbid suspension, 10^{-2} and 10^{-4} dilutions are prepared. The drug plates and one control quadrant are each inoculated with 0.1 ml of the 10^{-2} dilution, and the second control quadrant is inoculated with 0.1 ml of the 10^{-4} dilution.

Occasionally, it is not possible to obtain a smooth suspension of cells, especially if the culture is quite old. In that case it may be necessary to allow the microorganisms to grow in Dubos Tween-albumin broth until a turbid suspension is obtained. This broth culture should be treated the same way as a direct suspension of colonies.

Incubation and Reading. The inoculated plates are placed, medium side down, in individual polyethylene plastic bags and sealed. They are then incubated in an atmosphere of 5% to 10% carbon dioxide at 35°C. The plates are examined weekly for three weeks with the aid of a dissecting microscope, using 30 to 60 × magnification and transmitted light. The amount of growth is recorded as 4+ if confluent growth is seen; 3+ if innumerable, nearly confluent colonies are seen; 2+ if 100 to 200 colonies are seen; and 1+ if 50 to 100 colonies are seen. If fewer than 50 colonies are seen, the actual count is recorded.

In most cases it is easy to estimate the proportion of resistant colonies as greater than or fewer than 1% of the control population. That is to say, if the growth on a drug quadrant clearly exceeds the growth on the second dilution control (a 1:100 dilution of the inoculum), then more than 1% of the population is resistant. Often, resistant strains may be reported before the three-week incubation period is completed, i.e., as soon as clearly recognizable growth occurs on drug-containing quadrants as well as on the control medium. Since resistant colonies sometimes appear a little more slowly on the drug quadrant than on the control plate, tests indicating susceptibility cannot be reported before three weeks of incubation has been completed. On rare occasion, resistant colonies may not appear until four or five weeks of incubation, and thus the plates may be held for two weeks after the final three-week report is issued. Occasionally, a follow-up report may be required to describe those strains that produce resistant colonies in the last two weeks.

For the test to be valid, the inoculum should be dense enough to provide from 50 to 100 colonies on the second control quadrant. A lighter inoculum does not permit an accurate estimate of the cell population, and a denser inoculum might similate drug resistance because of growth of spontaneously occurring drug-resistant mutants.

REFERENCES

1. Griffith, M., M. L. Barrett, H. L. Bodily, and R. M. Wood. 1967. Drug susceptibility tests for tuberculosis using drug impregnated disks. Am. J. Clin. Pathol. 47: 812-817.
2. Runyon, E. H., A. G. Karlson, G. P. Kubica, and L. G. Wayne. 1974. Mycobacterium. In *Manual of Clinical Microbiology*, 2d ed. E. H. Lennette, E. H. Spaulding, and J. P. Truant (Eds.). American Society for Microbiology, Washington, D. C. pp. 148-174.

3. Vestal, A. L. 1973. Drug susceptibility tests. In *Procedures for the Isolation and Identification of Mycobacteria*. Public Health Service. Publication No. 1995. U.S. Government Printing Office, Washington, D. C. pp. 77-94.
4. Wayne, L. G., and I. Krasnow. 1966. Preparation of tuberculosis susceptibility testing mediums by means of impregnated discs. Am. J. Clin. Pathol. *45:* 769-771.

Section IV
AGAR
DIFFUSION
TESTS

Chapter 13

AGAR DIFFUSION: GENERAL CONSIDERATIONS

Agar diffusion techniques are commonly used for measuring the concentration of antimicrobic in serum or other body fluids or for determining the susceptibility of a particular microorganism. In principle, the techniques are quite simple: nutrient agar plates are inoculated in a standard manner and then the antimicrobic or unknown serum samples are applied to the agar surface in some type of reservoir. After an appropriate period of incubation, there is a circular zone of inhibited growth around the reservoir as a result of the antimicrobic, which has diffused into the surrounding agar. All other variables being equal, the size of the zone of inhibition is proportional to the log of the concentration of antimicrobic in the reservoir, a fact that has permitted the development of fairly sophisticated assay procedures for determining the concentration of antibiotic in serum or other solutions. If the amount of drug in the reservoir is held constant and all other variables are standardized, the size of the zone of inhibition is a measure of the degree of susceptibility of the test organism; i.e., the more susceptible the test strain, the larger the zone of inhibition. This fact has permitted the development of fairly sensitive, accurate methods for determining antimicrobic susceptibility. These methods are described in the following chapters.

163

USE OF DRIED FILTER-PAPER DISCS

In the mid-1940s, several investigators independently conceived of the idea that penicillin assay tests could be simplified by using filter-paper discs that had been soaked in antibiotic solutions.[9] Because of its simplicity, this idea was soon adapted to the susceptibility test, but it was limited by the need for preparing and storing stock solutions of the antimicrobics being tested. A significant improvement was made when it was found that the discs could be prepared in advance and stored under dry conditions until needed.[16] Commercially prepared dried discs soon became available for susceptibility testing and were readily accepted by most clinical laboratories. The vast majority of susceptibility tests now being performed in the United States are carried out with an agar diffusion technique, using dried filter-paper discs prepared by one of three commercial suppliers.

In the earlier work, the discs were designated according to the *concentration* (μg or IU/ml) of drug in the solution used for their preparation. The *potency* or *content* of the disc (amount of drug in each disc) obviously would not be the same as the concentration in the stock solution. The amount of drug contained by each disc depends on the volume retained by the disc after dipping and draining of excess fluid, which, in turn, depends upon the quality of the paper.

In a large-scale operation, discs are usually prepared by soaking sheets of filter paper in solutions of the antimicrobic. The sheets may be stamped in advance to designate the type of antimicrobic. The drug-soaked sheets of paper are then passed through a wringer to eliminate excess fluid and then allowed to dry in a well-ventilated area. Round discs, ¼ inch (6.35 mm) in diameter, are then stamped out on a punch press and transferred to storage vessels. The concentration of antimicrobic in this solution can be varied according to the amount retained by the particular batch of filter paper (usually determined gravimetrically). According to FDA standards,[8,13] the paper should weigh 30 mg ± 4 mg/cm,[2], and should absorb 2.5–3 times its own weight in water. No two batches of paper are absolutely identical, and thus the concentration of antimicrobic in the stock solution needs to be adjusted occasionally to give discs of uniform potency. Capillarity of the paper is not always homogeneous, and so the liquid may be absorbed unevenly. Consequently, there is some variation in the potency of discs stamped from the same sheet of filter paper, but with good manufacturing practices it is possible to produce discs that perform within very narrow tolerance limits.

On a smaller scale, very satisfactory discs may be prepared with ¼ inch (6.35 mm) diameter high-grade filter-paper discs (Schleicher and Schuell No. 740E). The discs are laid on an aluminum or stainless-steel wire mesh that is supported so as to allow circulation of air above and below the discs. Each disc is then charged with 0.02 ml of the appropriate‚ standard stock solution, using a suitably accurate micropipette. The discs are allowed to dry in circulating air or under vacuum. They are then transferred to an appropriate vessel and refrigerated in a desiccator. If the discs are to be held longer than one week, the desiccators may be stored in a freezer (–20°C or under)—especially if the discs contain one of the penicillins or cephalosporins. The performance of each batch of discs prepared in this way should be checked to avoid any adverse effects that may result from foreign materials in the filter paper or from the solvents used to prepare the drug solutions.

The discs currently available from commercial sources are generally quite satisfactory for susceptibility testing. This was clearly not the case some 20 years ago, when susceptibility testing was in its infancy.[2,3,18] Because of the poor quality of discs available at that time and because of the absence of well-standardized techniques, many investigators seriously questioned the reliability of disc diffusion testing altogether. Even today, the disc diffusion technique suffers from its past reputation. Many laboratorians still fail to appreciate the need for carefully standardized, controlled techniques. A better understanding of the agar diffusion technique and an appreciation of the consequences of deviating from the standardized methods can result from a review of some rather theoretical concepts concerning the dynamic forces influencing the formation of zones of inhibition. The following discussion is based largely upon the experimental work of Cooper and Linton.[4,5,6,14] Although most of their work was done with an agar diffusion procedure that differs significantly from the disc-plate technique under consideration, the principles Cooper and Linton established are generally applicable to this somewhat more complex testing system.[12,15]

DYNAMICS OF ZONE FORMATION

Once an agar diffusion test is initiated, two dynamic events proceed simultaneously. First, the antimicrobic diffuses into the surrounding medium, producing a gradually changing gradient of concentrations. At the same time, the microorganisms begin to metabolize, and after the initial lag phase, growth proceeds at a logarithmic rate. Early in the course of these events, the position of the zone of inhibition is determined and can be observed as soon as uninhibited growth becomes visible.

Antimicrobic Diffusion. When a dried filter-paper disc is applied to the surface of an inoculated agar medium, water is absorbed from the agar medium and the antimicrobic in the disc is dissolved. The concentration of drug at that point depends upon the volume of water absorbed and the amount of drug in the disc. The antimicrobic in solution then diffuses into the agar medium. At first, diffusion proceeds in three dimensions, but it soon becomes essentially two dimensional when the concentration in the depth of the agar approaches that at the surface. With very thin agar layers, outward diffusion proceeds more rapidly and thus the zones are somewhat larger.[1,7] During the first few hours of diffusion, the *concentration* of antimicrobic within the agar medium at the edge of the disc is relatively high and diminishes sharply at increasing distances from the disc. As diffusion progresses, the slope of the concentration gradient levels off, resulting in a broader gradient of decreasing concentrations within the agar medium (Fig. 13-1). With

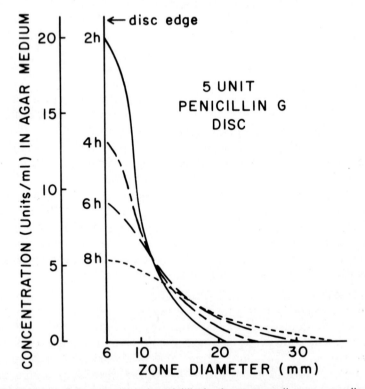

Figure 13-1. Concentration of penicillin in the agar medium surrounding a 5 unit disc after two, four, six, and eight hours of incubation (Data adapted from I. Hoette and A. P. Struyk. 1958. J. Lab. Clin. Med. *51:*643.)

continued diffusion, the amount of drug in the reservoir decreases, thus lessening the concentration gradient upon which diffusion depends.

The rate of diffusion through an agar gel depends upon the concentration of drug in the reservoir, the size and shape of the antimicrobic molecule, the viscosity of the agar gel, the temperature, and with some agents, the ionic content of the medium, and so on. For a given antimicrobic, the rate of diffusion through a given medium under controlled test conditions may be determined experimentally and expressed as a constant (diffusion coefficient). Under standardized test conditions, the distance reached by a particular concentration of an antimicrobic within a given period of time is proportional to the amount of antimicrobic in the reservoir.

Critical Concentration. A zone of inhibition is formed when a critical concentration of drug (that amount that is just capable of inhibiting microbial growth under the test conditions) reaches, for the first time, a density of growing cells too large for it to inhibit. The size of the zone of inhibited growth depends upon the time during which the critical inhibitory concentration can diffuse into the agar medium before a particular density of cells is reached. This, in turn, depends upon the diffusion coefficient of the drug and the concentration of drug applied to the reservoir. This critical concentration of drug can be determined experimentally and may be expressed by the general formula

$$\ln m' = \ln m_0 \ \frac{x^2}{4\,D T_0}$$

where $\ln m'$ = natural logarithm of the critical concentration

$\ln m_0$ = natural logarithm of the concentration of drug applied to the agar surface

x^2 = square of the distance between the reservoir and the edge of the zone of inhibition

D = diffusion coefficient for the antimicrobic under study, in the test medium and at the temperature of the test system

T_0 = critical time at which point the position of the zone of inhibition is determined

The m' may be determined by simultaneously testing several different concentrations of antimicrobic against the test organisms under standardized conditions. With constant conditions of inoculation, temperature, media, and timing of the experiment, $4 D T_0$ is a constant factor. The logarithm ($\log_e$ or $\log_{10}$) of m_0 plotted against x^2 should give a straight line, except for values of x less than 3 mm. Deviation from linearity with very small zones is to be expected because of the movement of water and salts between the antibiotic solution and the agar medium. By extrapolation, the concentration at the intercept (where $x^2 = 0$) may be determined; it is referred to as m', or the critical concentration, i.e., the concentration below which no zone of inhibition is formed. The m' is a useful measure of the susceptibility of the test organism and is usually related to but not identical to the MIC as measured by dilution techniques that involve somewhat different test conditions.

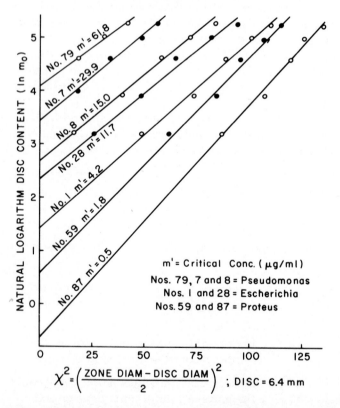

CARBENICILLIN

Figure 13-2. Estimation of critical concentrations of carbenicillin (m' values) for seven bacterial strains tested against 25-, 50-, 100-, 150-, and 200-µg discs. Each point represents the mean of 14 values (duplicate tests from seven different laboratories). (From A. L. Barry et al. 1976. J. Infect. Dis. in press.)

For example, data from a recent collaborative study concerning carbenicillin susceptibility tests[1a] are displayed in Figure 13-2. Each strain was tested in duplicate by seven different laboratories, using discs containing 200, 150, 100, 50, and 25 μg of carbenicillin. The mean zone size calculated for each disc potency was plotted against the natural logarithm of the disc content, and the critical concentration (m′) was calculated by regression analysis. At the same time, agar dilution tests were performed in four separate laboratories. Since three laboratories performed duplicate tests, seven MIC determinations were available for each strain. Table 13-1 lists the minimal, maximal, and modal MIC, which is compared to the m′ calculated from the agar diffusion data. Over a broad range of concentrations, the calculated m′ values may be compared to the agar dilution MICs, which varied by one or two doubling dilutions. In this particular set of experiments, the calculated m′ tended to be somewhat lower than the modal MIC value. Inhibitory

Table 13-1. Carbenicillin Agar Diffusion m′ Values and Agar Dilution MICs Determined as Part of a Multi-center Collaborative Study

	Culture Number	Critical Conc. (m′)*	Agar Dil. MICs† Mode	Agar Dil. MICs† Min.–Max.
		Inhibitory Concentrations (μg/ml)		
Klebsiella	#13	63.2	64	64 – 256
	#14	56.3	64	64 – 256
Pseudomonas	# 2	67.3	128	64 – 256
	#79	61.8	128	64 – 128
	# 6	35.1	32	32 – 64
	# 7	29.9	48	32 – 128
	# 9	19.7	32	16 – 32
	# 8	15.1	32	16 – 32
Escherichia	#28	11.7	8	8 – 16
	# 1	4.2	8	2 – 8
	# 7	2.8	4	≤ 1 – 4
Proteus	#59	1.8	2	≤ 1 – 4
	#52	1.4	≤ 1	≤ 1 – 1
	#87	0.5	≤ 1	≤ 1 – 8

Source: Adapted from A. L. Barry et al. 1976. J. Infect. Dis. (in press).

* Calculated m′ values based on 14 separate agar diffusion tests performed in 7 laboratories, each using 25, 50, 100, 150, and 200 μg carbenicillin discs (Fig. 13-2).

† MICs based on 7 separate series of tests performed in 4 different laboratories, all using the same testing procedure.

concentrations determined by agar diffusion and by standard dilution techniques should be comparable, within the limits of variability inherent in the two types of procedures.

Since the m' is independent of the variable DT_0, it presents a useful experimental method for studying the relationship between an antimicrobic and the test medium. For example, Figure 13-3

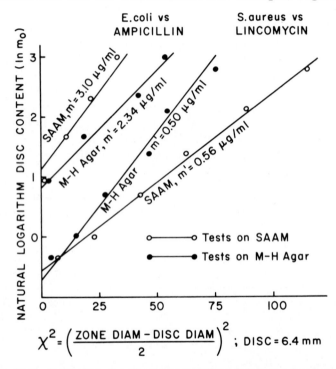

Figure 13-3. Estimation of critical concentrations (m') in the Synthetic Amino Acid Medium (SAAM) of Hoeprich et al.[10] compared to the m' in Mueller-Hinton (M-H) agar. Each value represents the mean of triplicate tests. (From A. L. Barry and L. J. Effinger. Unpublished data.)

summarizes the results of a study comparing the relative activity of ampicillin and lincomycin in Mueller-Hinton agar and in the synthetic amino acid medium (SAAM) of Hoeprich et al.[10] Although the two media produced markedly different zone sizes with high-content discs, the m' calculated from tests on the two media did not differ enough to explain the discrepancies in zone sizes. In the synthetic medium, the activity of ampicillin against *Escherichia coli* was reduced slightly, but not enough to explain the differences in mean zone sizes on the two media. The critical concentrations of lincomycin against *Staphylococcus aureus* on the two media were nearly identical although zones on the synthetic medium were significantly larger than those on Mueller-Hinton agar. Pre-incubation experiments (estimates of the critical time) suggest that the larger zone sizes seen with *E. coli* on M-H agar or with *S. aureus* on SAAM are related to a slightly prolonged growth rate rather than to an interaction between the antimicrobics and agar medium.

Although the m′ is independent of the variables DT_0, the slope of the line obtained by testing different concentrations varies with the rate of diffusion (D) and the time (T_0) required before the position of the zone is determined. This provides a convenient method for comparing the rates of diffusion of two or more related antimicrobic agents. A standard microorganism may be tested under controlled conditions against several concentrations of each of the drugs being studied. When all tests are performed at the same time, the variable T_0 should be a constant, and thus the slope of the line reflects the rate of diffusion of the different drugs. The intercept reflects the relative activity (m′) of the different drugs against the test organism. If the slopes of the regression lines demonstrate similar diffusion coefficients for related drugs, one can justify a direct comparison of zone diameters obtained with discs containing different, related agents. An example of such a study is shown in Figure 13-4.

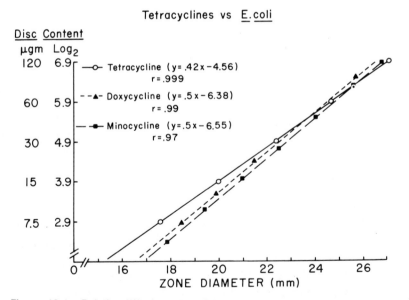

Figure 13-4.   Relative diffusion rates of three tetracyclines as estimated by plotting disc content against zone diameter. Each value represents the mean of triplicate tests. (From A. L. Barry and R. A. Lasner. Unpublished data.)

Critical Time. As mentioned above, the position of the zone of inhibition is determined at the point when the critical concentration of drug reaches for the first time a density of growing cells too large for it to inhibit. The critical time (T_0) can be determined experimentally by testing a susceptible microorganism under controlled conditions with a single concentration of drug, applied at different intervals after incubation has been initiated. When the antimicrobic is added at the same time that incubation is started, the position of the zone edge is determined after a critical time (T_0). If the microorganism is allowed to grow for h hours before the drug is added, the time of diffusion will be reduced to T_0-h and the zone should be smaller. By plotting the period of pre-incubation (h) against the zone of inhibition (x^2), a straight-line relationship should be seen for a given concentration of drug. By extrapolation, the line may be extended to the point where it intercepts at $x^2 = 0$. At that point, h equals T_0, the critical time at which the edge of the zone is formed and which may be expressed by the formula

$$T_0-h = x^2/4D \ln (m_0/m')$$

Where T_0 = critical time

$\quad\quad\quad$ h = hours of pre-incubation

$\quad\quad\quad$ x^2 = zone size squared

$\quad\quad\quad$ D = diffusion coefficient of the antimicrobic

$\ln (m_0/m')$ = natural logarithm of the concentration of drug in the reservoir divided by the critical concentration (m')

The critical time is independent of the concentration of antimicrobic in the reservoir; it expresses the rate of growth at a time when the antimicrobic is diffusing most rapidly through the agar medium. It is the time required for the microorganism to reach a critical cell mass.

Critical Population. After inoculation, the test organisms immediately begin to grow, passing through the early phases of the growth cycle. After an initial lag phase, the microorganisms enter into the logarithmic phase of growth, and multiplication then proceeds rapidly. Eventually the point is reached when a mass of cells has grown too large to be inhibited by the critical concentration of drug and growth can proceed more rapidly than additional drug can be built up by diffusion from the reservoir. This growth then proceeds to eventually become visible, demarcating the edge of the zone of inhibition. The relationship between critical time (T_0) and growth of the microorganism may be expressed by the formula

$$T_0 = L + G \log_2 (N'/N_0)$$

Where L = lag time

  G = generation time

  N′ = critical population at critical time (T_0)

  N_0 = number of viable cells at time 0 (inoculum density)

From this relationship it is clear that the critical time (T_0) is determined by the size of inoculum and rate of growth of the test organism. The density of the inoculum is an extremely important variable that can and must be controlled in order to obtain reliable results. The growth rate of the test strains is influenced by the inoculum size and by the nutritive capacity of the test media. A medium that supports unusually rapid growth of the test organism is not necessarily desirable because that will succeed only in reducing the sizes of the zones of inhibition. In the other extreme, tests on minimally nutritional media or tests with microorganisms that display unusually slow rates of growth tend to give exceptionally larger zones of inhibition. The growth rate of different strains is not readily controlled in the ordinary susceptibility test, and, for that reason, most diffusion techniques have been standardized for testing only the more common rapid-growing bacterial pathogens. They cannot be used routinely for testing slow-growing microorganisms.

NATURE OF THE ZONE OF INHIBITION

The foregoing discussion is based on the assumption that in the presence of a decreasing gradient of drug concentrations, microbial growth is either completely inhibited or is not inhibited at all and thus the edge of the zone of inhibition is sharply demarcated. In practice, most antimicrobics produce a zone of "partial" inhibition, which, at times, may be very difficult to visualize. There is often a spectrum of responses to the decreasing gradient of drug concentrations, giving the type of zone edge depicted in exaggerated form in Figure 13-5. From the disc outward there may be a zone of complete inhibition, surrounded by a ring of "partially inhibited" microbial growth, followed by a ring of "stimulated" growth set against a background of less profuse growth.

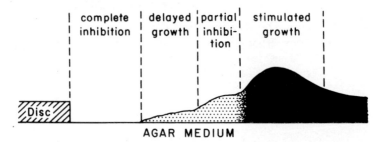

Figure 13-5. Exaggerated, diagrammatic view of microbial response to diminished concentrations of antimicrobic at the edge of a zone of inhibition.

The area of stimulated growth may be attributed more properly to a diminished growth in the background lawn because of an early depletion of nutrients available from the adjacent medium. Nutrients diffusing from the zone of inhibition are more readily available to those cells adjacent to the very edge and thus the total mass of growth is somewhat greater. This phenomenon is probably not related to a stimulating effect of sub-inhibitory concentrations of drug in the medium.

A band of partial inhibition is usually very narrow and probably represents a brief inhibition and eventual overgrowth that is often observed with sub-inhibitory concentrations of antimicrobics. One would expect to find inhibitory concentrations of drug inside this band of partial inhibition; thus, microbial growth should be completely inhibited. Occasionally, there is another very faint inner ring of delayed growth that represents viable cells initially inhibited by the concentration of drug at that point. This phenomenon can often be related to deterioration or inactivation of the drug, resulting in a delayed growth of those viable cells capable of surviving the initial inhibitory concentrations. This type of response is particularly striking in testing microorganisms that produce an extracellular enzyme, such as the penicillin β-lactamase of *Staphylococcus aureus*.

When the inoculum contains a small proportion of resistant variants, they eventually grow to produce visible colonies within a zone of inhibition. The initial inoculum of resistant cells may be relatively small and the resulting colonies may be small and slow in forming; they may fail to appear altogether in the area close to the disc, where drug concentrations are relatively high. To distinguish between secondary growth of resistant variants and delayed growth of susceptible survivors, one must subculture colonies from the area in question and repeat the test. This maneuver should increase the proportion of resistant variants and thus the repeat test should be more clear-cut. Of course, it is always necessary to distinguish contaminating microorganisms from resistant variants.

In testing the sulfonamides, a unique phenomenon may be observed. The microorganisms in the inoculum often contain sufficient intracellular reserve of pteroylglutamic acid, which must be exhausted before the competitive inhibition of *p*-aminobenzoic acid metabolism can be effective. Consequently, the cells undergo several generations before inhibition of growth can occur. If the inoculum is very light and the test medium free of sulfonamide antagonists, the result of this phenomenon of early growth is usually not visible since the metabolites are exhausted before the critical population of cells is obtained.

Microorganisms capable of swarming growth, e.g., *Proteus mirabilis* and *P. vulgaris*, often produce zones of inhibition that are initially clear and sharply defined. However, with further incubation and continued diffusion of the drug, inhibited growth from the outer ring is capable of swarming inward, thus obliterating the edge of the inhibitory zone. With an excessive amount of surface moisture, other types of microorganisms may spread into the zone of inhibition in a similar fashion. This phenomenon is not as significant a problem when the inoculum is applied as a pour plate or a seeded agar layer as it is when a swabbing or flooding method is used for inoculation.

FACTORS INFLUENCING THE SIZE OF INHIBITION ZONES

From the foregoing outline it should be clear that a variety of technical factors may influence the size of the zone of inhibition. Some factors may affect the results in several ways. The more important variables that are readily subject to experimental control are discussed in the following paragraphs.

Inoculum Density. The size of inoculum is probably the most important single variable that influences the zone of inhibition. The size of the zone of inhibition is not determined until a critical cell mass is obtained. With a small inoculum, more time is required to reach this cell mass, and thus the critical concentration of drug can diffuse further and the zone of inhibition is larger. A larger inoculum tends to give a smaller zone, and if the inoculum density exceeds the critical cell mass, the critical time for the zone size to be determined is equal to the lag time, which, in turn, is diminished with an extremely heavy inoculum. For that reason, susceptible strains may fail to produce any zone of inhibition with an extremely heavy inoculum, especially if a relatively low-content disc is being applied. On the other hand, relatively resistant strains may produce fairly large zones of inhibition if an extremely light inoculum is applied.

The effect of inoculum size is particularly profound when testing microorganisms that produce drug-inactivating enzymes. For example, penicillin β-lactamase–producing strains of *Staphylococcus aureus* may provide relatively large zones of inhibition around penicillin discs when a very light inoculum is applied. Rather slight increases in inoculum density result in a reduction of the size of the zone of inhibition disproportionately greater than that seen with nonpenicillinase-producing strains. That may be related to the fact that although the individual cells are susceptible to the action of the penicillin, they are protected by their ability to produce penicillinase enzymes. With a small inoculum, the penicillin may be capable of inhibiting the growth before the microorganism can produce enough enzyme to inactivate the drug. Each increase in inoculum density is accompanied by an increase in the amount of constitutive enzyme and, thus, by a marked shift in the apparent ability of the microorganism to grow in the presence of the penicillin. Once multiplication is initiated, induction of the extracellular β-lactamase results in further inactivation of the drug, and any viable cells surviving the initial action of the penicillin may then initiate growth.

Composition of the Agar Medium. The agar medium influences the zone size by (1) its effect on the activity of the antimicrobic, (2) its influence on the rate of diffusion of the antimicrobic, and (3) its effect on the growth rate of the test organism. Many of the factors that affect the activity of specific antimicrobics were described in Chapter 4. The rate of diffusion of the drug is determined to some extent by the concentration of agar and the concentration of various ions in the medium. The nutritive capacity of the agar may have a significant influence on the length of the lag phase and generation time for the microorganism under test. Nutritionally deficient media produce much larger zones of inhibition, probably because a prolonged lag phase is required before growth can be initiated.

Temperature of Incubation. Susceptibility tests are normally incubated at 35°C (34°-36°C) for optimal growth of most human pathogens. A single plate placed on the metal shelf of an incubator takes one hour to warm to within 1°C of the incubator temperature, but, if the plates are piled five deep, the center plate takes up to four hours to reach the same temperature.[5,15] Since the rate of growth of the test strain may be prolonged at lower incubation temperatures, a delay in reaching optimal temperatures extends the time required for the critical concentration of cells to be reached.

Consequently, plates in the center of a stack produce slightly larger zones than those on the top or bottom, because the critical concentration of antimicrobic has more time to diffuse. In contrast, most antimicrobics diffuse more slowly with lower temperatures, thus complicating the effect exerted by the temperature during the first few hours of incubation. For accurate comparative studies, great care must be taken to obtain uniform heating of the test plates. The test plates should be prewarmed for the same period of time and should be placed singly on the same incubator shelf—but such extreme precautions are normally not necessary for routine susceptibility tests.

Most bacterial pathogens are not greatly influenced by slight changes in incubation temperature, but the temperature is extremely important when testing methicillin against *S. aureus*. The methicillin-resistant portion of a population of staphylococci is more readily detected at a lower temperature (30°C). Although the susceptible portion of the heterogenous population will grow adequately at 35° to 37°C, the minority population of resistant cells may not be detected at temperatures of 36°C or greater, whereas they usually grow at 35°C or less.[17]

Finally, some antimicrobics are relatively unstable at ordinary incubator temperatures. In most cases, a significant amount of deterioration does not occur until after the position of the zone of inhibition is determined. Deterioration of drug would have to be extremely rapid to reduce the definite zone edge, which is formed at the critical time (T_0). However, once the position of the zone of inhibition is determined, inactivation of the drug progresses, followed by the gradual development of an inner ring of delayed growth. This delayed growth may be obvious enough to give the appearance that the zone size is diminishing as incubation continues or that slow-growing resistant variants are beginning to emerge with prolonged incubation.

Timing of Disc Application. After the test plates have been inoculated, they are often allowed to dry for a defined period of time before the discs are applied. This drying step is essential to prevent leaching of the antimicrobic from the disc into the layer of surface moisture that may be left immediately after swabbing or flooding a freshly prepared agar medium. In practice, when a large number of test plates are being put up, the time lapse between inoculation and disc application may vary considerably from plate to plate. Some procedures require a specific period of prediffusion at room temperature after the discs are applied, to provide additional time for the antimicrobic to diffuse through the agar gel before the critical concentration is reached. It is extremely important to standardize the time so that each test plate receives the same treatment.

Incubation Time.   Since the position of the zone of inhibition is determined within the first few hours of incubation, the zones of inhibition may be measured as soon as microbial growth becomes visible. With many common bacterial pathogens, definite zones of inhibition can be observed within five to six hours of inoculation. However, the zones often become smaller with further incubation because of changes in the character of the growth at the zone edge resulting from (1) the appearance of delayed growth or (2) better visualization of partially inhibited growth or (3) delayed appearance of resistant variants. Occasionally, the zones appear to increase in size because of changes in the character of the growth at the zone edge or because of actual lysis of the initial growth within the inner ring of the zone.

Potency of Antimicrobic Discs.   The amount of drug in the disc is proportional to the size of the zone of inhibition but, fortunately, rather large changes in disc content are required to effect a major shift in the zone size; with many drugs, a 50% loss of activity results in only a 2- or 3-mm decrease in zone diameter (Fig. 13-4). For the sake of standardization, the discs must be of uniform potency, and every possible precaution must be taken to avoid deterioration of the antimicrobic during storage of the discs.

Depth of Agar Medium.   Since diffusion of the antimicrobic is initially three dimensional, the thicker the agar plate the smaller the amount of drug available to diffuse laterally and, consequently, the smaller the zone of inhibition. With very thin plates, slight changes in agar depth influence zone sizes dramatically, but as the volume of the agar medium increases, the effect of minor changes in agar depth becomes almost negligible.[1,7] For susceptibility testing, the depth of the agar medium should be held at approximately 4 mm. A reasonable degree of caution in filling the plates can readily control this source of variability; extreme precision is not necessary.

From the discussion above it should be obvious that the size of the zone of inhibition can be influenced by a number of variables, most of which can be controlled rather accurately if well-standardized procedures are carefully performed. Under these conditions, the amount of day-to-day variability is relatively small, and the disc diffusion test is truly an accurate analytical procedure, not just a qualitative screening procedure.

REFERENCES

1. Barry, A. L., and G. D. Fay. 1973. The amount of agar in antimicrobic disk susceptibility test plates. Am. J. Clin. Pathol. *59:* 196-198.
1a. Barry, A. L., et al. 1976. Inter- and intra-laboratory variability in susceptibility tests with *Pseudomonas aeruginosa* and *Enterobacteriaceae.* J. Infect. Dis. in press.
2. Branch, A., D. H. Starkey, and E. E. Power. 1959. The international situation with regard to the use of discs for antibiotic sensitivity tests. In *Antibiotics Annual 1958–1959.* Medical Encyclopedia, Inc., New York. pp. 833-835.
3. Branch, A., D. H. Starkey, K. C. Rodgers, and E. E. Power. 1955. Experience with controlling antibiotic sensitivity tests in Department of Veterans Affairs hospital laboratories in Canada. In *Antibiotics Annual 1954–1955.* Medical Encyclopedia. Inc. New York. pp. 1125-1132.
4. Cooper, K. E. 1963. The theory of antibiotic inhibition zones. In *Analytical Microbiology.* F. Kavanagh (Ed.). Academic Press, New York. pp. 1-86.
5. Cooper, K. E., and A. H. Linton. 1952. The importance of the temperature during the early hours of incubation of agar plates in assays. J. Gen. Microbiol. 7: 8-17.
6. Cooper, K. E., A. H. Linton, and S. N. Sehgal. 1958. The effect of inoculum size on inhibition zones in agar media using staphylococci and streptomycin. J. Gen Microbiol. *18:* 670-687.
7. Davis, W. W., and T. R. Stout. 1971. Disc plate method of microbiological antibiotic assay, I. Factors Influencing Variability and Error. Appl. Microbiol. 22: 659-665.
8. Federal Register. 1961. Antibiotics intended for use in the laboratory diagnosis of disease. Fed. Regist. *26:* 2596.
9. Garrod, H. P., and N. G. Heatley. 1944. Bacteriological methods in connection with penicillin treatment. Br. J. Surg. *32:* 117-124.
10. Hoeprich, P. D., A. L. Barry, and G. D. Fay. 1970. Synthetic medium for susceptibility testing. Antimicrob. Agents Chemother. *10:* 494-497.
11. Hoette, I., and A. P. Struyck. 1958. A modified method for evaluation of clinical usefulness of antibiotics. J. Lab. Clin. Med. *51:* 638-653.
12. Humphrey, J. H., and J. Lightbown. 1952. A general theory for plate assay of antibiotics with some practical applications. J. Gen. Microbiol. 7: 129-143.
13. Kirshbaum, A., J. Kramer, and B. Arret. 1960. The assay and control of antibiotic discs. Antibiot. Chemother. *10:* 249-258.
14. Linton, A. H. 1958. Influence of inoculum size on antibiotic assays by the agar diffusion technique with *Klebsiella pneumoniae* and streptomycin. J. Bacteriol. 76: 94-103.
15. Linton, A. H. 1961. Interpreting antibiotic sensitivity tests. J. Med. Lab. Technol. *18:* 1-20.
16. Morley, D. C. 1945. A simple method for testing the sensitivity of wound bacteria to penicillin and sulfathiazole by use of impregnated blotting paper discs. J. Pathol. Bacteriol. *57:* 379-382.
17. Thornsberry, C., J. Q. Caruthers, and C. N. Baker. 1973. Effect of temperature on the *in vitro* susceptibility of *Staphylococcus aureus* to penicillinase-resistant penicillins. Antimicrob. Agents Chemother. *4:* 263-269.
18. Wright, W. W. 1974. FDA actions on antibiotic susceptibility discs. In *Current Techniques for Antibiotic Susceptibility Testing.* A. Balows (Ed.). Charles C Thomas, Springfield, Ill. pp. 26-46.

Chapter **14**

DIFFUSION TEST PROCEDURES

The fundamental principles of agar diffusion procedures were described in the previous chapter. From that discussion, it should be obvious that well-standardized, carefully controlled techniques are needed to obtain optimal results. In 1968, Bauer and co-workers[8] published the details of a carefully standardized technique that can be controlled adequately. With this method, the inoculum is prepared by adjusting the turbidity of an actively growing broth culture to match that of a $BaSO_4$ standard. Because this critical step is often thought to be too cumbersome for routine work, more expedient but less reliable modifications have been made without substantiation of adequacy. This situation led Barry and co-workers[4] to develop an agar overlay method that is significantly easier to read and simpler to perform. The diffusion technique currently recommended by the FDA[14, 15] and described as an approved standard of the National Committee for Clinical Laboratory Standards[18] is a slight modification of the technique described by Bauer et al. in 1968. The agar overlay method of Barry et al. is recognized formally as an acceptable alternative method for standardizing the inoculum when testing the commonly isolated rapid-growing bacterial pathogens, such as *Staphylococcus aureus*, the *Enterobacteriaceae*, and *Pseudomonas aeruginosa*. These two test procedures are the only methods currently recognized as acceptable procedures. They are described in detail in a later section of this chapter.

180

APPLICATIONS AND LIMITATIONS OF DIFFUSION TESTS

Antimicrobic susceptibility tests should be performed only with those clinical isolates thought to be contributing to an infectious process that warrants chemotherapy and provided that the microorganism's susceptibility cannot be predicted from a knowledge of its identity. In practice, susceptibility tests are most often indicated when the causative microorganism has been identified as a species known to be capable of exhibiting resistance to commonly used antimicrobic agents, e.g., *Staphylococcus* sp., the *Enterobacteriaceae*, and *Pseudomonas* sp. Susceptibility tests are rarely necessary when the infection is due to a microorganism that is invariably susceptible to an effective drug, e.g., most pathogenic streptococci and *Neisseria* sp. are predictably susceptible to one or more highly effective antimicrobics. When the nature of the infection is not clear, and the specimen contains mixed growth of normal flora in which the microorganisms probably bear little relationship to the infectious process being treated, susceptibility tests are often wasteful or grossly misleading.

If carefully performed, disc diffusion tests reliably classify most test strains into resistant or susceptible categories (Chapters 2, 15). However, certain limitations inherent in the disc diffusion procedure must be fully appreciated.

1. The disc diffusion technique has been standardized primarily for microorganisms that grow rapidly on the standard medium (rapid growth occurs if an endpoint can be easily determined within an 18 to 24 hour period). Beyond that time, diffusion of the antimicrobic or inactivation of the drug may give erroneous results, and thus microorganisms with a prolonged generation time cannot be tested accurately by the disc diffusion method.

2. The disc test does not measure the bactericidal activity of a drug.

3. Combinations of two or more antimicrobial agents cannot be assayed with the standard disc diffusion technique, with the exception of sulfonamide-trimethoprim.

4. Microorganisms classified as resistant by the disc diffusion technique should not be affected by concentrations of a drug that are normally obtained in the serum of patients, but exceptionally high doses of a drug may bring about a cure. Infections at sites where a drug is concentrated might also respond even though the etiologic agent is categorized as resistant.

Broth or agar dilution techniques should be employed for more exact definition of the concentration required to inhibit growth or to exert a lethal effect, to study combinations of antimicrobics, or to test slow-growing or nutritionally fastidious microorganisms. In short, the disc diffusion technique generally provides the type of information required to treat infections involving those bacterial pathogens most commonly encountered in clinical specimens. Alternative procedures are needed when exceptional situations arise.

SELECTION OF ANTIMICROBICS FOR ROUTINE DIFFUSION TESTING

Because of the ever-increasing number of antimicrobial agents available, the selection of drugs to be tested on a routine basis may be difficult. To simplify the routine test, the number of drugs must be sharply limited. On the other hand, each laboratory report should include information about all the drugs that may be of interest to the physicians of the particular institution. The laboratory director is constantly faced with requests to add more and more drugs to their routine protocol because the agents reported as part of the routine susceptibility tests profoundly influence the use of different chemotherapeutic agents within the institution. After consultation with the appropriate clinical staff, a laboratory may elect to withhold a toxic or ineffective drug from routine testing in order to limit use of the agent within the institution. Antimicrobics other than those appropriate for use in therapy may be tested to provide epidemiologic information and taxonomic data. However, to avoid misleading information, routine reports to physicians should include only those drugs appropriate for therapeutic use.

Certain drugs should not be tested because there is good reason to believe that the results of *in vitro* tests may be irrelevant. For example, *in vitro* tests with methenamine mandelate should not be performed because the activity of this drug *in vivo* depends on the attainment of a urinary pH of 5 or less, and *in vitro* test conditions bear no relationship to the situation in the urine—the only possible site of antibacterial activity in the patient.[25]

Antimicrobics are usefully classified into groups with similar modes of action; drugs within each group often demonstrate complete or partial cross-resistance. Although there may be significant differences in the pharmacologic properties of closely related drugs, there is little value in testing more than one representative from each group. The FDA has recognized specific class discs, which were selected to represent such groups of related antimicrobics.[14] The agents listed in Table 14-1 should fulfill the basic requirements for routine diffusion testing in most clinical laboratories. Additional antimicrobics should be available for use when special problems of the individual patient are to be taken into account.

AGAR DIFFUSION PROCEDURES

The essential principles of the currently recommended agar diffusion disc methods are as follows:

Agar Medium. Both methods have been standardized with

Table 14-1. Suggested Battery of Antimicrobics for Routine Susceptibility Testing of Clinical Isolates

Gram-Positive Cocci		Gram-Negative Bacilli	
Staphylococcus sp.	*Enterococcus*	*Enterobacteriaceae*	*Other*
1. Penicillin G	1. Penicillin G	1. Ampicillin	1. Gentamicin
2. Oxacillin	2. Ampicillin	2. Cephalothin	2. Carbenicillin
3. Cephalothin	3. Cephalothin	3. Kanamycin	3. Polymyxin B
4. Erythromycin	4. Erythromycin	4. Gentamicin	4. Kanamycin†
5. Clindamycin	5. Chloramphenicol	5. Polymyxin B	5. Chloramphenicol†
6. Chloramphenicol	6. Tetracycline	6. Tetracycline	6. Tetracycline†
7. Tetracycline		7. Chloramphenicol	7. Sulfonamide* †
8. Gentamicin		8. Nitrofurantoin*	
9. Kanamycin		9. Nalidixic Acid*	
		10. Sulfonamide*	

* Only for isolates from urinary tract infections.

† Indicated for testing pseudomonads and other nonfermentative bacilli, excluding *P. aeruginosa*.

Mueller-Hinton agar. The reasons for selecting this medium and various control parameters were covered extensively in Chapter 4. The agar medium should be dispensed into plastic petri plates on a level horizontal surface so as to give a uniform depth of approximately 4 mm; this requires approximately 60 ml of medium in 150-mm plates, or approximately 25 ml in 100-mm plates.[2,13] After the medium has been allowed to cool to room temperature, it should be stored in a refrigerator (from 2°-8°C). If the plates are to be stored for more than from five to seven days, they should be wrapped in plastic to minimize evaporation. Just before use, the plates should be placed in an incubator (35°C) with lids ajar until excess surface moisture evaporates (usually about 30 minutes). There should be no droplets of moisture on the surface of the medium nor on the petri plate cover. With the agar overlay method of inoculation, the plates must be warmed to room temperature, but the surface need not be dried before inoculation.

Storage of Antimicrobic Discs. Antimicrobic cartridges containing filter-paper discs specifically certified for susceptibility testing are generally supplied in separate containers, packaged so as to insure appropriate anhydrous conditions. They should be stored under refrigeration (from 2°-8°C) or preferably "frozen" at-14°C or lower until needed. Discs containing drugs that belong to the penicillin or cephalosporin families should always be kept "frozen" to insure maintenance of their potency.[13,18] However, a small working supply may be held in a refrigerator (from 2° to 8°C) with a desiccant for as long as one week. Unopened containers should be removed from the refrigerator or freezer one or two hours before the discs are to be used and allowed to equilibrate to room temperature before being opened. This procedure minimizes the amount of condensation that would occur if warm room air reached the cold containers. If a disc-dispensing apparatus is used, it should be fitted with a tight cover and supplied with an adequate indicating desiccant. It also should be allowed to warm to room temperature before being opened. When not in use, the dispensing apparatus should always be kept covered and refrigerated. Only those discs that have not reached the manufacturer's expiration date should be used.

Inoculation of Test Plates—Standard Method. The currently recommended standard method (the "Kirby-Bauer" technique) is employed as follows:

1. Select at least four or five well-isolated colonies of the same morphologic type from an agar plate culture. Touch the top of each colony with a wire loop and transfer the growth to a tube containing 4 to 5 ml of a suitable broth medium, such as soy bean casein digest broth.

2. Allow the broth culture to incubate at from 35° to 37°C until it achieves or exceeds the turbidity of the standard described below (usually from two to eight hours).

3. Adjust the turbidity of the actively growing broth culture with sterile saline or broth so as to obtain a turbidity visually comparable to the turbidity standard described below. To perform this step properly, there must be an adequate source of light and reading should be made against a white background with a contrasting black line to aid in the visual comparison. The modified Rh typing view box described by Stemper and Matsen[21] facilitates standardization of cultures by this technique. When time does not permit the development of a turbid broth culture, colonies can be suspended directly into a small volume of saline, which is then further diluted until the turbidity matches that of the $BaSO_4$ standard.[6] The inoculum suspension should not be allowed to stand any longer than from 15 to 20 minutes before the plates are inoculated.

4. The turbidity standard is prepared by adding 0.5 ml of 0.048 M $BaCl_2$ (1.175% w/v $BaCl_2 \cdot 2 H_2O$) to 99.5 ml of 0.36 N H_2SO_4 (1% v/v). This is equal to half the density of a No. 1 MacFarland standard. The tubes are tightly sealed and stored in the dark at room temperature. Unless the standard is contained in heat-sealed glass tubes,[7,24] it should be replaced at least once every six months. A fresh standard should be prepared more frequently if there is any evidence (as indicated by quality control procedures) that deterioration may have occurred. The turbidity standard must be agitated vigorously on a mechanical vortex shaker just before each use.

5. Within 15 minutes of adjusting the density of the inoculum suspension, a sterile cotton swab on a wooden applicator is dipped into the standardized suspension and the excess inoculum removed from the swab by rotating several times with a firm pressure on the inside wall of the test tube above the fluid level.

6. Inoculate the dried surface of a Mueller-Hinton agar plate by streaking the swab over the entire sterile agar surface. Repeat this streaking procedure two more times, rotating the plate approximately 60 degrees each time so as to insure an even distribution of inoculum. If the plate is satisfactorily streaked, the zones of inhibition are uniformly circular and there is a uniform confluent, or almost completely confluent, lawn of growth. Replace the plate top and allow three to five minutes (no longer than 15 minutes) for any excess surface moisture to be absorbed before applying the drug-impregnated discs.

Alternative Agar Overlay Method of Inoculation. A more efficient, acceptable alternative method for inoculating the test plates is employed as follows:

1. Select four or five isolated colonies of the same morphologic type from an agar plate culture and prepare a visibly turbid suspension in 0.5 ml of brain-heart infusion broth in a 13-by-100-mm tube. To avoid changes due to evaporation during storage of this small volume of broth it is transferred aseptically into sterile tubes on the day it is to be used.

2. Incubate the small-volume broth cultures in a 35° to 37°C water bath or heating block for at least four hours (no longer than eight hours). By this time, maximal growth should have occurred.

3. Transfer a 0.001-ml calibrated loopful of the well-mixed broth culture to 9.0 ml of a 1.5% aqueous solution of agar that has been melted and held from one to eight hours in a 45° to 50°C heating block (in 16-by-125-mm screw-cap tubes). The caps are tightened after the agar is melted, and unused tubes are discarded at the end of the day to avoid changes in agar concentration due to evaporation.

4. Quickly mix the seeded agar by gentle inversion and then spread over the surface of a 150-by-15-mm petri plate containing Mueller-Hinton agar (4 mm in depth). To facilitate this procedure, the plates are brought to room temperature before attempting to spread the thin layer of seeded agar.

5. Allow the inoculated plate to stand from three to five minutes undisturbed on a flat and level surface and then apply susceptibility discs as described below.

Application of Discs. Within 15 minutes after the plates are inoculated, apply antimicrobic-impregnated discs to the surface of the inoculated plates either with a mechanical dispenser or by hand with sterile forceps. With sterile forceps or needle tip gently press down each disc to insure complete contact with the agar surface. The spatial arrangement of the discs must be such that they are no closer than 15 mm from the edges of the plate and far enough apart to prevent overlapping of zones of inhibition, i.e., no more than 24 mm from center to center. Generally, this limits the number of discs that can be placed on a single plate to 12 or 13 on a 150-mm plate, or only four or five on a 100-mm plate. Since some diffusion of drug is almost instantaneous, a disc should not be moved once it has come in contact with the agar surface.

Incubation of Test Plates. The plates are then inverted and placed in a 35°C incubator within 15 minutes after the discs are applied; any longer delay before incubation allows excess prediffusion of the antimicrobic. Incubation in an environment of increased CO_2 is to be avoided because the CO_2 will alter the surface pH enough to affect the antimicrobial activity of some agents. For standard reference work, careful control of incubator temperature is critically important. The individual plates should be evenly dispersed over the incubator shelf without stacking so that each plate reaches incubator temperatures at approximately the same time.

Reading and Interpretation. After 16 to 18 hours of incubation, the plates are examined and the diameter of the zones of complete inhibition is measured to the nearest whole millimeter with a sliding caliper, ruler, or template prepared for this purpose. When an unsupplemented medium is used, the measuring device is held on the back of the petri plate, which is illuminated with reflected light. Similar systems using transmitted light may also be used if comparable zone sizes are obtained with quality-control strains. Zones on a blood-containing medium are measured at the agar surface. The end-point by all reading systems is complete inhibition of growth as determined visually, ignoring faint growth or tiny colonies that can be detected only under very close scrutiny. Large colonies growing within the clear zone of inhibition may represent resistant variants or a mixed inoculum and may require re-identification and retesting. With sulfonamide or sulfonamide-trimethoprim mixtures, the microorganisms may grow through several generations before inhibition occurs. In this instance, slight growth (20% of the uninhibited growth) is disregarded, and the margin of heavy growth is measured.[9] With *Proteus* sp., a veil of swarming growth is disregarded and the margin of heavy growth is measured. In clinically urgent situations, preliminary readings can be obtained often within five or six hours of inoculation, but the plates should always be re-incubated and, if necessary, a corrective report issued after a full 16 to 18 hours have elapsed.[6,8]

The zone diameters for individual antimicrobics are translated into prefixed susceptible, intermediate or resistant categories by referring to an interpretative table. The interpretations for the antibiotics in Table 14-2 are those presently recommended by the FDA[14,15] and by the National Committee for Clinical Laboratory Standards.[18] They are supplemented by recommendations from other sources for the non-antibiotic drugs. The approximate MIC correlates that were used for defining the susceptible and resistant categories described by these zone standards are also listed in Table 14-2. Three significant changes in the zone-size recommendations included in Table 14-2 are currently under consideration. They are:

1. Consolidation of the penicillin and ampicillin interpretative criteria. Those given for ampicillin against staphylococci and against *Enterobacteriaceae* and enterococci would apply to both antimicrobics, as would the category "other organisms" listed for penicillin. This change would take into account the high systemic and urine levels of penicillin that are achieved with doses appropriate for treating gram-negative and enterococcal infections.[5]

2. A shift in the gentamicin breakpoint for susceptibility to a zone diameter of 15 mm or more, and the establishment of an intermediate category of 13 to 14 mm. This has been proposed because a few strains of *Pseudomonas* sp. have been encountered with zones of 13 or 14 mm and agar dilution MICs as high as 12.5 μg/ml.

3. Zone standards for oxacillin and nafcillin 1-μg discs against staphylococci. These have been recommended because the two agents are more stable than methicillin and are just as effective as methicillin—or more effective—in detect-

ing resistance to the penicillinase-resistant penicillins. The recommended standards for both 1-μg discs are (1) resistant = 10 mm or less, (2) intermediate = 11 to 12 mm, and (3) susceptible = 13 mm or more.

It is to be anticipated that some agreed-upon changes in the interpretative chart will result from such proposals and that additional changes will occur from time to time as further knowledge is gained and new agents become available. Because the selection of MIC and zone-size breakpoints requires a somewhat arbitrary, best-judgment decision (Chapters 2, 15), some differences of opinion are bound to arise whenever independent groups develop interpretive standards. Until the differences listed above are resolved, the zone-size standards in Table 14-2 are recommended for routine use.

The MIC correlates listed in Table 14-2 are related to blood levels usually expected with frequently used dose schedules, or to urine levels in the case of nitrofurantoin or nalidixic acid.

SPECIAL PRECAUTIONS

Methicillin-Resistant Staphylococcus aureus. Strains of *S. aureus* that display hetero resistance to the β-lactamase-resistant penicillins and cephalosporins can be detected readily by testing with methicillin, oxacillin, or nafcillin discs at temperatures of 35°C but often not at 37°C.[11,12,23] If incubators cannot be controlled at 35°C, separate tests with one of these agents only should be made on segments of Mueller-Hinton agar plates incubated at 30°C. Diffusion tests with these strains often fail to indicate resistance to cloxacillin and cephalothin although dilution tests show it to exist. Thus strains proved to be resistant to methicillin, oxacillin, or nafcillin should be considered potentially resistant to the whole group of penicillinase-resistant penicillins and cephalosporins; the clinician should be alerted to this fact. False reports of methicillin resistance may result from deterioration of methicillin discs.[12] Attention to the recommendations given above for disc storage and quality control should avoid this difficulty.

Gentamicin. As discussed in earlier chapters, gentamicin susceptibility of *Pseudomonas aeruginosa* is highly dependent upon the concentration of cations in the medium, especially of magnesium and calcium cations. Most batches of Mueller-Hinton agar are satisfactory for routine testing and interpretation by the criteria given in Table 14-2. However, it is important to use a control strain of *P. aeruginosa* to detect errors from this source of variability. The establishment of an intermediate category of interpretation for gentamicin could help avoid serious interpretative errors that might occur from minor technical variations in cation concentrations.

Table 14-2. Zone-Diameter Interpretive Standards and Approximate MIC Correlates

Antimicrobial Agent	Disc Content	Zone-Diameter (mm): Nearest Whole mm Resistant	Intermediate	Susceptible	Approximate MIC Correlates Resistant	Susceptible
Ampicillin*—when testing gram-negative enteric organisms and enterococci	10 µg	≤ 11	12–13	≥ 14	≥ 32 µg/ml	≤ 8 µg/ml
Ampicillin*—when testing staphylococci and penicillin G-susceptible micro-organisms	10 µg	≤ 20	21–28	≥ 29	≥ 32 µg/ml Penicillinase†	≤ 0.2 µg/ml
Ampicillin*—when testing Hemophilus species	10 µg	≤ 19	—	≥ 20	—	≤ 2.0 µg/ml
Carbenicillin—when testing Proteus species and Escherichia coli	100 µg‡	≤ 17	18–22	≥ 23	≥ 32 µg/ml	≤ 16 µg/ml
Carbenicillin—when testing Pseudomonas aeruginosa	100 µg‡	≤ 13	14–16	≥ 17	≥ 250 µg/ml	≤ 125 µg/ml
Cephalothin‡	30 µg	≤ 14	15–17	≥ 18	≥ 32 µg/ml	≤ 10 µg/ml
Chloramphenicol	30 µg	≤ 12	13–17	≥ 18	≥ 25 µg/ml	≤ 12.5 µg/ml
Clindamycin	2 µg	≤ 14	15–16	≥ 17	≥ 2 µg/ml	≤ 1 µg/ml
Colistin	10 µg	≤ 8	9–10	≥ 11	—¶	—
Erythromycin	15 µg	≤ 13	14–17	≥ 18	≥ 8 µg/ml	≤ 2 µg/ml
Gentamicin	10 µg	≤ 12	—	≥ 13	≥ 6 µg/ml	≤ 6 µg/ml
Kanamycin	30 µg	≤ 13	14–17	≥ 18	≥ 25 µg/ml	≤ 6 µg/ml
Methicillin‖—when testing staphylococci	5 µg	≤ 9	10–13	≥ 14	—	≤ 3 µg/ml

Neomycin	30 μg	≤ 12	13–16	≥ 17	—	≤ 10 μg/ml
Penicillin G #—when testing Staphylococci	10 units	≤ 20	21–28	≥ 29	Penicillinase†	≤ 0.1 μg/ml
Penicillin G #—when testing other micro-organisms	10 units	≤ 11	12–21**	≥ 22	≥ 32 μg/ml	≤ 1.5 μg/ml
Polymyxin B	300 units	≤ 8	9–11	≥ 12	≥ 50 units/ml¶	—
Streptomycin	10 μg	≤ 11	12–14	≥ 15	≥ 15 μg/ml	≤ 6 μg/ml
Tetracycline††	30 μg	≤ 14	15–18	≥ 19	≥ 12 μg/ml	≤ 4 μg/ml
Vancomycin	30 μg	≤ 9	10–11	≥ 12	—	≤ 5 μg/ml
Sulfonamides‡‡	250 or 300 μg	≤ 12	13–16	≥ 17	≥ 350 μg/ml	≤ 100 μg/ml
Trimethoprim-sulfamethoxazole‡‡	1.75 μg 23.25 μg	≤ 10	11–15	≥ 16	≥ 200 μg/ml	≤ 35 μg/ml
Nitrofurantoin‡‡	300 μg	≤ 14	15–16	≥ 17	≥ 100 μg/ml	≤ 25 μg/ml
Nalidixic Acid‡‡	30 μg	≤ 13	14–18	≥ 19	≥ 32 μg/ml	≤ 12 μg/ml

* Class disc for ampicillin, hetacillin, and amoxicillin.

† Resistant strains of S. aureus produce penicillinase.

‡ Class disc for cephalothin, cephaloridine and cephalexin, cephazolin and cephapirin.

¶ Colistin and polymyxin B diffuse poorly in agar, and thus the accuracy of diffusion tests is less than that found with other antimicrobics and MIC correlates cannot be calculated reliably from regression analysis.

‖ Class discs for penicillinase-resistant penicillins.

Class disc for benzylpenicillin, phenoxymethyl penicillin, and phenethicillin.

** Intermediate category includes some microorganisms, such as enterococci, and certain gram-negative bacilli that may cause systemic infections treatable with high dosages of benzylpenicillin but not of phenoxymethyl penicillin or phenethicillin.

†† Class disc for tetracyclines.

‡‡ Used only for testing isolates from urinary tract infections.

Polymyxins. The accuracy of the disc test is dependent upon the adequate diffusion of the antimicrobic under study—and the polymyxins (B and E) diffuse very poorly. Although resistance is significant, it is important to confirm susceptibility by a dilution test if one of these agents is to be used for systemic therapy.

Sulfonamide-resistant Neisseria meningitidis. To provide a guide for prophylactic therapy and to provide useful epidemiologic information, *N. meningitidis* may be tested for sulfonamide resistance. Most isolates are capable of growing adequately on Mueller-Hinton agar without supplements, and thus a slight modification of the standard method may be used.[10] The most difficult phase of this test procedure involves the preparation of a standardized inoculum. After overnight incubation of the test strains on Mueller-Hinton agar, growth is suspended in 10 ml of Mueller-Hinton broth so as to obtain a minimally visible turbidity (with an optical density of from 0.04 to 0.06 at 625 nm). A sterile cotton swab is dipped into the suspension, excess fluid removed from the swab by gentle pressure against the inside of the test tube, and the surface of a Mueller-Hinton agar plate inoculated immediately by swabbing the entire surface in four different axes. For these tests, plastic petri dishes 10 cm in diameter should contain 19 ml of Mueller-Hinton agar. Once inoculated, the surface of the agar should be allowed to dry for three to five minutes, and then a single 300-μg sulfathiazole disc is applied to the center of the plate with sterile forceps and gently pressed onto the agar surface. Uninverted plates are incubated for 18 hours at 35°C in a candle jar. The diameter of the zone of inhibition is then determined by observing the plates against a dark background. When a slight film of growth occurs within an otherwise obvious zone of inhibition, the clearly distinguishable outer margin of the inhibitory zone is measured. Strains producing zones of 40 mm or greater are considered susceptible (MIC less than 1 mg/100 ml), whereas resistant strains produce zones of inhibition 36 mm or less, leaving an intermediate, equivocal category of from 37 to 39 mm (Chapter 15).

Anaerobic Susceptibility Tests. Although routine susceptibility testing of anaerobic or other fastidious microorganisms is not recommended, there are circumstances in which such testing might be relevant to proper management of the clinical situation. In serious infections with a single pathogen, e.g., endocarditis or brain abscess, the antimicrobial susceptibility of the individual isolate should be determined by a broth or agar dilution procedure (Chapters 5, 6). Those laboratories not equipped to do adequately controlled dilution studies might be able to contribute useful information by performing a disc diffusion test. Although testing procedures have not yet been standardized for anaerobic bacteria, the following method is widely applicable and reasonably practical for testing most of the rapid-growing anaerobes commonly encountered in human clinical specimens.[3,16,22]

The test strain is first grown overnight in thioglycolate medium without indicator (BBL-135C), which is supplemented with hemin (5 μg/ml) before autoclaving and $NaHCO_3$ (1 mg/ml) and vitamin K_1 (0.1 μg/ml) after autoclaving. The inoculum is then standardized by adjusting the turbidity of the broth culture to match that of a No. 1 MacFarland standard—giving about 10^7 to 10^8 viable cells per ml. Tests are performed on Brucella agar (Pfizer) containing 5% defibrinated sheep blood and vitamin K_1 (10 μg/ml). The plates are dried in a 35°C incubator for one hour prior to use and then inoculated with the swabbing procedure. A maximum of four antimicrobic discs are applied to each 10-cm petri plate. Zones of inhibition are measured after 42 to 48 hours of incubation at 35°C in Gas-Pak jars. The results are then interpreted by referring to the zone standards in Table 14-3.

Direct Inoculation with Clinical Specimens. In some clinical situations, reliable results are needed more quickly than can be obtained with the standard methods described above. Earlier results can be made available by inoculating the test plates directly with clinical materials rather than waiting until isolated colonies are available. However, specimens that are likely to contain members of the normal microbiota may yield grossly misleading results with direct susceptibility tests since one is not allowed the opportunity to select the potential pathogens for which susceptibility

Table 14-3. Zone-Diameter Interpretive Standards for Estimating Qualitative Susceptibility of Rapidly Growing Unidentified Anaerobes According to the Method of Sutter et al.[22]

Antimicrobial Agent	Disc Content	Zone Diameter (mm): Nearest Whole mm		
		Resistant	Equivocal	Susceptible
Chloramphenicol	30 μg	$\leqslant 14$	15–20	$\geqslant 21$
Clindamycin	2 μg	$\leqslant 8$	9–14	$\geqslant 15$
Penicillin G*	10 U	$\leqslant 12$	13–28	$\geqslant 29$
Tetracycline	30 μg	$\leqslant 15$	16–28	$\geqslant 29$

* With *F. varium* and *F. mortiferum*, penicillin zones are based on 80% inhibition of growth.

testing is most relevant. Furthermore, the size of the inoculum cannot be standardized and controlled when the clinical specimen is applied directly to the test plates. For these reasons, the direct susceptibility test should be considered to be, at best, a poorly controlled, unstandardized technique with which major errors of interpretation must be expected. However, this procedure might provide useful information in a clinical emergency. When the specimen contains more than one type of microorganism, the reliability of the direct susceptibility test is markedly diminished.[6,20] Table 14-4 summarizes the results of one series of tests with 517 urine specimens, comparing directly inoculated susceptibility tests to indirect standardized tests with pure culture isolates. Discrepant results (usually with one or two antimicrobics) were obtained with 37% of the 517 specimens. One or more major discrepancies (resistant with one method, susceptible with the other) were seen with

Table 14-4. Interpretation of Disc Diffusion Susceptibility Tests Inoculated Directly with Urine Specimens as Compared to Indirect Tests with Pure Culture Isolates

Microorganism(s) Isolated (All Specimens >10⁵ Bacteria/ml)	Total Number of Specimens Tested	Number of Specimens with One or More Discrepancies*	
		Minor	Major
One microorganism: Total	396	50 (13%)	68 (17%)
Escherichia coli	232	20	37
Klebsiella-Enterobacter	55	11	9
Enterococci	41	9	6
Proteus mirabilis	40	6	8
Pseudomonas aeruginosa	20	4	6
Other	8	0	2
Two microorganisms: Total†	100	15 (15%)	46 (46%)
Enterococcus + another†	46	6	19
P. mirabilis + another†	35	4	18
P. aeruginosa + another†	20	3	11
Other combinations	13	3	6
Three microorganisms: Total	21	2 (9%)	10 (48%)
Total specimens	517	67 (13%)	124 (24%)

SOURCE: A. L. Barry et al. 1973. Am. J. Clin. Pathol. *59:*694.

* Major discrepancies: one or more drugs resistant with one method, susceptible with the other. Minor differences involve an intermediate zone with one method but not the other.

† 14 specimens are included under two subtotals (four with enterococcus and *P. mirabilis*, five with *P. mirabilis* and *P. aeruginosa*, and five with *P. aeruginosa* and enterococcus).

46% of those specimens containing more than one microorganism but with only 17% of those specimens in which a single microorganism predominated. No one drug in particular was involved more than another, nor could the direction of the error be predicted in advance. Although the direct approach has some practical value, it should never be used as a substitute for the delayed standardized methods now available. In urgent clinical situations, the directly inoculated susceptibility plates can provide useful preliminary information, which may be reported as such, to be modified as necessary the following day, after standardized tests have been performed.

EVALUATION OF ALTERNATIVE DISC
DIFFUSION TECHNIQUES

There is little question that the currently recommended methods can be improved upon in a number of ways. Microbiologists may be tempted to modify the standardized methods for their own convenience without determining whether the interpretive zone standards still apply. Laboratory workers unable to evaluate alternative methods adequately are to be discouraged from deviating from the described standard methods. Without sufficient supportive data, deviations from the described techniques must be considered unsatisfactory. The type of information required to evaluate alternative techniques properly is outlined below to serve as a guide for those who wish to propose other methods.

A series of recent clinical isolates must be tested by the proposed method in parallel with the currently recommended technique, recording the observed zone diameters around all relevant antimicrobic discs. For each agent, the diameter observed on both types of test plates can then be plotted against one another and a regression analysis used to determine the degree of correlation. If a significant difference exists, the regression line may be used to suggest new interpretive standards for the proposed method. The number of tests necessary for statistically significant results is difficult to determine, but generally a minimum of from 100 to 150 selected isolates is needed, provided that zone diameters are evenly distributed and that there are no points along the line where excessive numbers of data points are accumulated.

The accuracy of the disc diffusion method must be evaluated by a correlation between inhibitory zone diameters and minimal inhibitory concentrations (broth or agar dilution tests). Selected strains obtained during the comparative study described in the previous paragraph should be further tested by a broth or agar dilution technique in parallel with repeated disc diffusion tests. These studies should include all strains with which the interpretation of the two disc diffusion techniques disagree and all strains that give intermediate zone sizes. In addition, a few strains that are susceptible by both methods and a few strains that are resistant by both disc methods should be tested by antimicrobic dilution techniques. For each drug, at least 50 microorganisms should be tested in this manner.

The precision of the proposed diffusion method must also be documented. On at least 50 different occasions, two or more control organisms should be tested by the standard reference procedure and by the new proposed alternative technique. The resulting data for each method can then be compared by calculating both the mean zone diameter and the standard deviation for each of the antimicrobic agents being tested. To be acceptable, the proposed technique must be capable of producing a standard deviation no greater than that of the recommended procedure and both should be well within the acceptable tolerance limits described in Chapter 16.

Such an evaluation requires a considerable investment of time and energy, and this should discourage those microbiologists who wish to modify standard procedures without seriously evaluating the consequences of the alterations thus introduced.

REFERENCES

1. Barry, A. L. 1974. The agar overlay technique for disc susceptibility testing. In *Current Techniques for Antibiotic Susceptibility Testing.* A. Balows (Ed.). Charles C Thomas, Springfield, Ill. pp. 17-25.
2. Barry, A. L., and G. D. Fay. 1973. The amount of agar in antimicrobic disc susceptibility test plates. Am. J. Clin. Pathol. 59:196-198.
3. Barry, A. L., and G. D. Fay. 1974. Evaluation of four disk diffusion methods for antimicrobic susceptibility tests with anaerobic gram-negative bacilli. Am. J. Clin. Pathol. 61:592-598.
4. Barry, A. L., F. Garcia, and L. D. Thrupp. 1970. An improved method for testing the antibiotic susceptibility of rapidly growing pathogens. Am. J. Clin. Pathol. 53:149-158.
5. Barry, A. L., and P. D. Hoeprich. 1973. *In vitro* activity of cephalothin and three penicillins against *Escherichia coli* and *Proteus* sp. Antimicrob. Agents Chemother. 4:354-360.
6. Barry, A. L., L. J. Joyce, A. P. Adams, and E. J. Benner. 1973. Rapid determination of antimicrobial susceptibility for urgent clinical situations. Am. J. Clin. Pathol. 59:693-699.
7. Bartlett, R. C., and M. Mazens. 1973. Analytical variability in the single disk antimicrobial susceptibility test. Am. J. Clin. Pathol. 59:376-383.
8. Bauer, A. W., W. M. M. Kirby, J. C. Sherris, and M. Turck. 1966. Antibiotic susceptibility testing by a standardized single disk method. Am. J. Clin. Pathol. 45:493-496.
9. Bauer, A. W., and J. C. Sherris. 1974. The determination of sulfonamide susceptibility of bacteria. Chemotherapy 9:1-19.

10. Bennett, J. V., H. M. Camp, and T. C. Eickhoff. 1968. Rapid sulfonamide disc sensitivity test for meningococci. Appl. Microbiol. *16:*1056-1060.
11. Churcher, G. M. 1968. A screening test for the detection of methicillin-resistant staphylococci. J. Clin. Pathol. *21:*213-217.
12. Drew, W. L., A. L. Barry, R. O'Toole, and J. C. Sherris. 1972. Reliability of the Kirby-Bauer disc diffusion method for detecting methicillin-resistant strains of *Staphylococcus aureus*. Appl. Microbiol. *24:*240-247.
13. Ericsson, H. M., and J. C. Sherris. 1971. Antibiotic sensitivity testing. Report of an international collaborative study. Acta Pathol. Microbiol. Scand. Sect. B, Suppl. 217.
14. Federal Register. 1972. Rules and regulations. Antibiotic susceptibility discs. Fed. Regist. *37:*20525-20529.
15. Federal Register. 1973. Rules and regulations. Antibiotic susceptibility discs: Correction. Fed. Regist. *38:*2576.
16. Kwok, Y. Y., F. P. Tally, V. L. Sutter, and S. M. Finegold. 1975. Disk susceptibility testing of slow-growing anaerobic bacteria. Antimicrob. Agents Chemother. *7:*1-7.
17. Matsen, J. M., and A. L. Barry. 1974. Susceptibility testing: Diffusion test procedures. In *Manual of Clinical Microbiology*, 2d ed. E. H. Lennette, E. H. Spaulding, and J. P. Truant (Eds.). American Society for Microbiology, Washington, D. C. pp. 418-427.
18. NCCLS Subcommittee on Antimicrobial Susceptibility Tests. 1975. *Performance Standards for Antimicrobial Disc Susceptibility Tests*. National Committee for Clinical Laboratory Standards. 771 E. Lancaster Ave., Villanova, Pa. 19085.
19. Ryan, K. J., F. D. Schoenknecht and W. M. M. Kirby. 1970. Disc sensitivity testing. Hospital Practice *5:*91-100.
20. Shahidi, A., and P. D. Ellner. 1969. Effect of mixed cultures on antibiotic susceptibility testing. Appl. Microbiol. *18:*766-770.
21. Stemper, J. E., and J. M. Matsen. 1970. Device for turbidity standardization of cultures for antibiotic sensitivity testing. Appl. Microbiol. *19:*1015-1016.
22. Sutter, V. L., Y. Y. Kwok, and S. M. Finegold. 1974. *In vitro* susceptibility testing of anaerobes: Standardization of a single disc test. In *Anaerobic Bacteria: Role In Disease*. A. Balows, R. M. Dehaan, V. R. Dowell, and L. B. Guze (Eds.). Charles C Thomas, Springfield, Ill. pp. 457-476.
23. Thornsberry, C., J. Q. Caruthers, and C. N. Baker. 1973. Effect of temperature on the *in vitro* susceptibility of *Staphylococcus aureus* to penicillinase-resistant penicillins. Antimicrob. Agents Chemother. *4:*263-269.
24. Washington, J. A., E. Warren, and A. G. Karlson. 1973. Stability of barium sulfate turbidity standards. Appl. Microbiol. *24:*1013.
25. Waterworth, P. M. 1962. A misapplication of the sensitivity test: Mandelamine discs. J. Med. Lab Technol. *19:*163-168.

Chapter 15

ESTABLISHMENT OF ZONE-SIZE INTERPRETIVE CRITERIA

The inverse relationship between the size of zone of inhibition and the minimal inhibitory concentration (MIC) is critically important to all agar diffusion techniques. When the test conditions are held reasonably constant, susceptibility tests with microorganisms of nearly comparable growth rates should display a linear relationship between the diameter of the zone of inhibition and the $\log_2$ of the MIC, as determined by standard dilution techniques. For each antimicrobial agent, a characteristic zone size : MIC relationship can be documented, thus permitting an approximation of the MIC from a given zone determination. Following the principles outlined in Chapter 2, it is possible to establish MIC breakpoints above which an organism should be considered resistant and an MIC below which the organism is classified as susceptible. With some drugs, there will be an intermediate category between these two breakpoints. Such MIC breakpoints are developed after considering (1) the pharmacokinetics of each antimicrobic, (2) the behavior of microorganisms of known clinical responsiveness or nonresponsiveness, and (3) the overall distribution of MICs and zone diameters with relevant clinical isolates. The very same principles may be applied in the development of zone-size interpretive criteria for agar diffusion susceptibility tests.

Figures 15-1 to 15-7 illustrate the type of data that can be collected with different drugs to document the relationship between zone diameters and MICs, using standardized methods and a fixed disc content. Figures 15-2 to 15-7 give agar dilution MICs and disc diffusion zone measurements determined for each strain in at least three different laboratories independently, as part of a large collaborative study reported in 1975.[10] The relationship between zone diameter and MIC may present (1) an even distribution of end-points over the more relevant range of drug concentrations (Figs. 15-1, 15-2), (2) a clear bimodal distribution of end-points, with a tendency for most genera to cluster at either end of the scale (Figs. 15-3, 15-4), or (3) a cluster of end-points in the susceptible range with virtually no distinct resistant population (Figs. 15-5, 15-6). Three different considerations must be taken into account in establishing zone-size interpretive criteria once the MIC breakpoints have been defined for separating the resistant and susceptible categories.

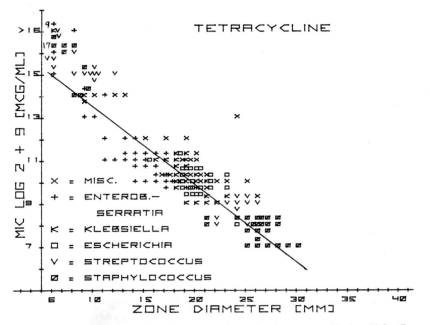

Figure 15-1. Tetracycline: 189 zones (30-μg discs) vs. agar dilution MICs. Regression formulas: Y = 17.11–0.36X; correlation coefficient, r = 0.90; N = 153 (36 tests with no zone of inhibition or with MICs outside the range of concentrations tested were excluded from the calculations). (From A. L. Barry. Unpublished data.)

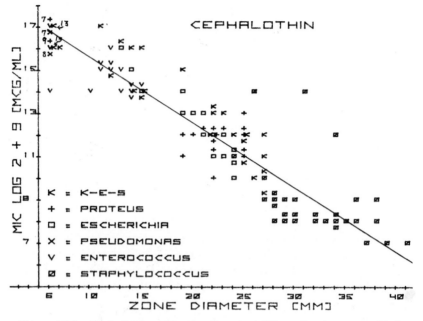

Figure 15-2. Cephalothin: 155 zone diameters (30-μg discs) vs. agar dilution MICs, as determined by three independent investigators. Regression formulas: Y = 18.65–0.30X; correlation coefficient, r = 0.89; N = 95 tests (60 tests with no zones were excluded from the calculations). The three *Staphylococcus* sp. with 25-to-35-mm zones but MICs of eight or 32 μg/ml (log$_2$ +9 = 12 or 14) were "methicillin"-resistant strains. (Data kindly provided by A. K. Knirsch.)

Regression Analysis. The linear correlation between MICs and zone sizes can be expressed mathematically by applying the formula of least squares to calculate the line of best fit (regression line). This approach is frequently misapplied, often to inappropriately distributed data. For an appropriate regression analysis, the test organisms must be selected to provide MICs that are fairly evenly distributed over a relevant range of concentrations and should include representatives of the common species of bacteria for which the antimicrobic agent might be used. In general, about 100 to 150 strains should be tested by a standard dilution technique and by a disc diffusion procedure. The data are then examined by plotting each MIC value against the corresponding zone diameter.[3]

A regression line is then calculated by the method of least squares, assuming that there is a straight-line relationship and neglecting the experimental error inherent in the MIC determination. In calculating a regression line, all MIC values above and below the actual concentrations tested and all disc tests showing no zone of inhibition should be excluded. Because the lines are intended for extrapolating ranges of MIC correlates from diffusion test results, the MICs may be plotted as the dependent variable (Y) and the zone diameters plotted as the independent variable (X). This provides a regression formula:

$$Y = a + bX$$

Where b = an expression of the slope of the line
a = the intercept (the theoretical Y value when X = O)

With this formula, it is possible to calculate an MIC correlate for a given zone diameter, based on studies with a relatively small collection of carefully selected bacterial isolates. A regression line can be quite misleading if calculated from data that fail to disperse evenly along the entire range of MIC values, as is often the case with some antimicrobic agents (Figs. 15-5 to 15-7).

Scatter Diagrams. When the distribution of end-points does not permit a regression analysis, the relationship of MIC to zone diame-

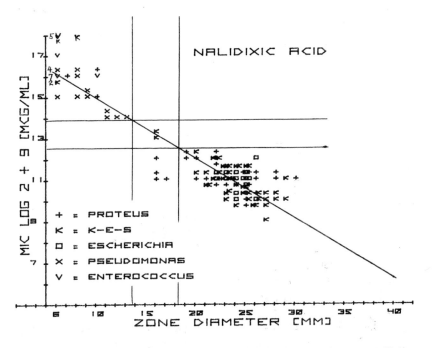

Figure 15-3. Nalidixic acid: 120 zone diameters (30-µg discs) vs. agar dilution MICs, as determined by three independent investigators. Regression formulas: Y = 17.44–0.28X; correlation coefficient, r = 0.90, N = 98 (22 tests with no zones of inhibition or MICs outside the range of concentrations tested were excluded from the calculations). A susceptible zone of 19 mm or more corresponds to an MIC ≤ 8 µg/ml, and a resistant zone of 13 mm or less corresponds to an MIC ≥ 32 µg/ml. (Data kindly provided by A. K. Knirsch.)

ter is best expressed as a simple scatter diagram in which MIC values are plotted against matching zone diameters. This approach is especially important when there is a broad distribution of zone diameters for a given MIC value, as when a very large unselected sample of microorganisms has been tested or when the MIC values are subject to rather pronounced experimental error.

Once MIC breakpoints have been selected, interpretive zone standards can be established by visually examining the scatter diagram. The "error rate-bounded" classification scheme of Metzler and DeHaan[5] has been proposed as a formal method for establishing zone-size interpretive standards from those scatter diagrams that do not permit regression line analysis. The method may be stated as follows: Let the maximal tolerable rate (% error) for false resistance be P_R and the maximal tolerable rate (% error) for false susceptible be P_s. Given a sample of N determinations of MICs and zone diameters, the maximal zone for the resistant category (Z_R) and the minimal zone for the susceptible category (Z_s) may be cho-

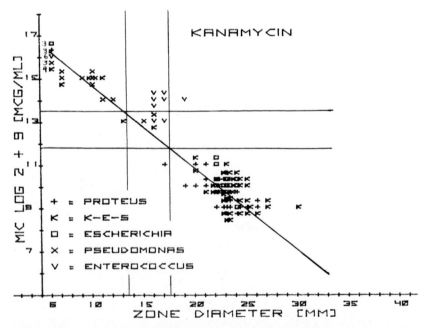

Figure 15-4. Kanamycin: 119 zone diameters (30-μg discs) vs. agar dilution MICs, as determined by three independent investigators. Regression formulas: Y = 18.54–0.38X; correlation coefficient, r = 0.93; N = 100 tests (19 tests with no zones of inhibition were excluded from the calculations). A susceptible zone of 18 mm or more corresponds to an MIC ≤ 4 μg/ml, and a resistant zone of 13 mm or less corresponds to an MIC ≥ 32 μg/ml. (Data kindly supplied by A. K. Knirsch.)

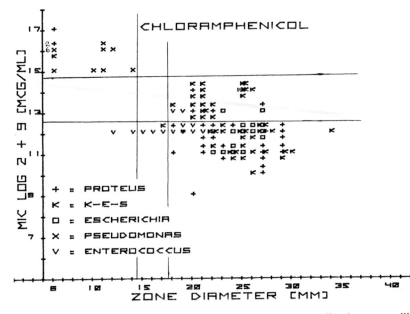

Figure 15-5. Chloramphenicol: 122 zone diameters (30-µg discs) vs. agar dilution MICs, as determined by three independent investigators. A regression line drawn through these data might be misleading (r = 0.55) because of a marked tendency for the end-points to cluster within the susceptible or intermediate category, whereas most resistant strains produce no zone of inhibition and are not included in the regression analysis. MIC breakpoints and established interpretive zone standards are drawn in to aid in the evaluation of these data. (Data kindly provided by A. K. Knirsch.)

sen so that (1) the number of strains falsely classified as susceptible is $P_s \times N$, (2) the number of strains classified as resistant is $P_R \times N$, and (3) the number of strains classified as intermediate is as small as possible. The latter consideration often influences the decision concerning what P_s and P_R values can be tolerated.

After the maximal tolerable rate of error is chosen, the breakpoints Z_R and Z_s can be determined by inspection of the scatter diagram as displayed in Figure 15-8. If the data are listed with the zone diameters ranked, then it is easy to progress from small to large zone diameters counting false resistance until the maximal tolerable rate of error (P_R) is reached. Likewise, one can go from a large zone diameter to a smaller zone diameter counting false susceptible tests until P_s is reached. The process is easily programmed for automatic computation, but this is rarely necessary.

This approach completely ignores the experimental error inherent in the MIC determinations. Furthermore, consideration of the pharmacologic properties of the antimicrobic under study requires

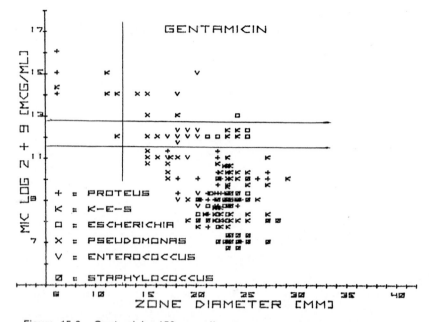

Figure 15-6. Gentamicin: 156 zone diameters vs. agar dilution MICs, as determined by three independent investigators. A regression line should not be applied to these data because of a poor correlation coefficient (r = 0.54). The currently recognized interpretive zone standard of 13 mm or more for susceptible is drawn in, along with MIC breakpoints of 16 μg/ml or greater for resistant and 4 μg/ml or less for susceptible. (Data kindly provided by A. K. Knirsch.)

the establishment of an intermediate MIC category. When an intermediate category is used, the error-rate–bounded scheme becomes a little more difficult but is still applicable. For example, in the above-mentioned example (Fig. 15-8) if the MIC for susceptible were 1.6 μg/ml or less and for resistant 12.5 μg/ml or greater, an MIC of 6.2 or 3.1 μg/ml would be considered intermediate and should give zones in the intermediate category. Misclassification of strains with intermediate MICs may be considered minor errors, whereas other erroneous categorizations are major errors. Zone-size breakpoints drawn by the rate-bounded method would still be appropriate provided that one could define the number of major and minor errors that could be accepted. Further examination of the scatter diagrams should be made to determine whether the zone-size breakpoints could be shifted slightly in order to decrease the range of zone diameters depicting the intermediate category without producing an excessive number of major errors in interpretation. To some extent, the final location of the zone-size breakpoint involves some degree of subjectivity and some best-judgment decisions. These breakpoints should be tested further by examining the overall distribution of zone sizes with a much larger collection of relevant clinical isolates, and, if necessary, minor adjustments may be made to separate populations that display a clear bimodal distribution of zone diameters.

Population Analysis. When a collection of isolates of one species tends to produce clusters of end-points at either end of the scale (i.e., either very large zones and low MIC values or very small zone sizes and relatively high MIC values), a regression analysis may not be appropriate. In that situation, interpretive schemes for disc tests with that species can be based on the characteristics of the two populations, provided that the MICs for the susceptible population bear a reasonable similarity to clinically obtainable blood levels. The resistant and susceptible populations might be defined best if each isolate were tested three or more times and for each strain the geometric mean MIC plotted against the arithmetic mean zone diameter, as shown in Figure 15-9. With such a clear bimodal distribution of MICs and zone diameters, it is possible to establish interpretive criteria by calculating the exact probability for correct

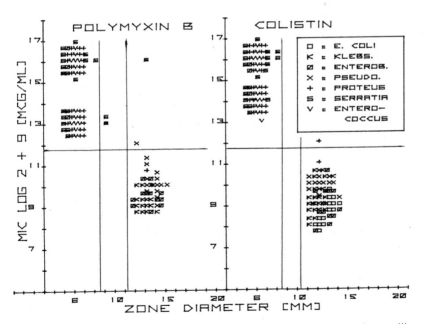

Figure 15-7. Polymyxins: Relationship between zone diameters and agar dilution MICs, as determined independently by three collaborating investigators. Valid regression analysis is not possible with these drugs. (Data kindly provided by A. K. Knirsch.)

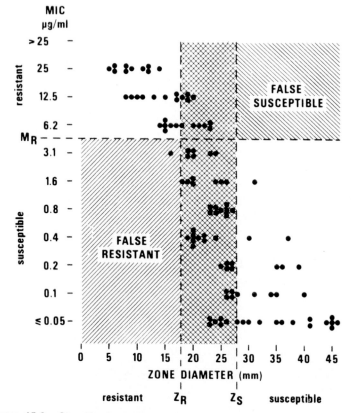

Figure 15-8. Classification scheme for zone diameters obtained by the error rate-bounded method. (From C. M. Metzler, and R. M. DeHaan. 1974. J. Infect. Dis. *130:* 589.)

or incorrect interpretation in the critical area between the populations of zone sizes.[2]

With some antimicrobics, clinical isolates present a clear unimodal distribution of susceptible strains with no resistant variant. In such cases, only one temporary zone standard can be established since none of the above-mentioned criteria are applicable for the establishment of a maximal zone size for the resistant population that might appear once the drug has received broad use.

THE INTERMEDIATE CATEGORY

With the above-mentioned considerations, one may establish a minimal zone of inhibition produced by susceptible strains and, with most drugs, a maximal zone of inhibition produced by resistant strains. Between these two values, there is an intermediate cate-

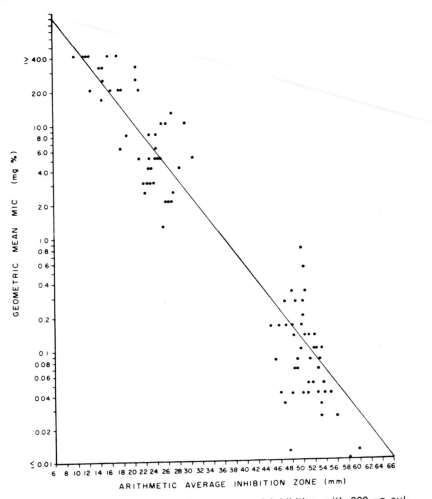

Figure 15-9. *N. meningitidis* MICs vs. zone of inhibition with 300-μg sulfathiazole discs. (From J. V. Bennett, H. M. Camp, and T. C. Eickhoff. 1968. Appl. Microbiol. *16:* 1058.)

gory, which is often referred to as *intermediate, indeterminate,* or *equivocal.* This category has two important functions: (1) it encompasses those strains with MICs that are neither clearly resistant nor fully susceptible. With some antimicrobics, a significant proportion of strains may be properly classified in this truly equivocal category, for which clinical response might be anticipated only when unusually high concentrations of drug can be achieved at the site of infection, and (2) it provides a "buffer zone" that minimizes the significance of minor technical variables that cannot be controlled completely with a practical working system. Because some variability is inherent in the procedure, the zone of inhibition produced by a given strain might vary from day to day by a matter of several millimeters. If that strain happens to produce a zone size at or near an interpretive zone breakpoint, the *interpretation* of the test varies from day to day. Consequently, when several isolates of the same strain are recovered from different specimens or from the same patient on different days, they may be reported as indeterminate or equivocal on some occasions and resistant or susceptible on other occasions. If the procedure is adequately controlled, the probability that the interpretation will vary from resistant to susceptible should be less than 1% with those strains giving mean zone diameters at or near an interpretive zone breakpoint.

If the disc test were modified by eliminating the intermediate category, and results reported only as resistant or susceptible, a significant number of major interpretive errors could occur as a result of relatively minor variations inherent in the procedure. Fortunately, with most drugs, the majority of isolates produce either very small or very large zones of inhibition, and equivocal, indeterminate test results are relatively uncommon. For that reason, minor variations in technique do not influence the interpretation of the majority of the tests. Strict standardization and quality control are particularly important when testing those few strains that produce zones of inhibition at or near the arbitrary breakpoints. When a disc test is reported to be equivocal and an alternative drug is not available for use, further study by a quantitative dilution procedure is clearly indicated. In practice, the majority of equivocal results involve drugs that are not being considered seriously for therapy of a particular patient.

REFERENCES

1. Bauer, A. W. 1964. The two definitions of bacterial resistance. In *Proceedings of the Third International Congress of Chemotherapy*. Stuttgart, Germany. pp. 484-500.
2. Bennett, J. V., H. M. Camp, and T. C. Eickhoff. 1968. Rapid sulfonamide disc sensitivity test for meningococci. Appl. Microbiol. 16:1056-1060.
3. Ericsson, H. M., and J. C. Sherris. 1971. Antibiotic sensitivity testing. Report of an international collaborative study. Acta Pathol. Microbiol. Scand. Sect. B, Suppl. 217.
4. Matsen, J. M., M. J. H. Koepcke, and P. G. Quie. 1969. Evaluation of the Bauer-Kirby-Sherris-Turck single-disc diffusion method of antibiotic susceptibility testing. Antimicrob. Agents Chemother. 9:445-453.
5. Metzler, C. M., and R. M. DeHaan. 1974. Susceptibility of anaerobic bacteria: Statistical and clinical considerations. J. Infect. Dis. 130:588-594.
6. NCCLS Subcommittee on Antimicrobial Susceptibility Tests. 1975. *Performance Standards for Antimicrobial Disc Susceptibility Tests*. National Com-

mittee for Clinical Laboratory Standards. 771 E. Lancaster Ave., Villanova, Pa. 19085.

7. Overman, S. B., D. W. Lambe, and J. V. Bennett. 1974. Proposed standardized method for testing and interpreting susceptibility of *Bacteroides fragilis* to tetracycline. Antimicrob. Agents Chemother. 5:357-361.

8. Petersdorf, R. G., and J. C. Sherris. 1965. Methods and significance of *in vitro* testing of bacterial sensitivity to drugs. Am. J. Med. 39:766-779.

9. Sherris, J. C., A. L. Roshad, and G. A. Lighthart. 1967. Laboratory determination of antibiotic susceptibility to ampicillin and cephalothin. Ann. N. Y. Acad. Sci. 145:248-265.

10. Thornsberry, C., T. L. Gavan, J. C. Sherris, A. Balows, J. M. Matsen, L. D. Sabath, F. Schoenknecht, L. D. Thrupp, and J. A. Washington II. 1975. Laboratory evaluation of a rapid, automated susceptibility testing system: Report of a collaborative study. Antimicrob. Agents Chemother. 7:466-480.

Chapter **16**

DISC DIFFUSION TESTS: QUALITY CONTROL

Many of the principles of an effective quality-control program were outlined in Chapter 8, and specific sources of variability with the agar diffusion technique were discussed extensively in Chapter 13. The following pages review some of the practical aspects of quality control for disc diffusion susceptibility testing in the clinical laboratory.

It must first be assumed that a well-standardized procedure has been adopted and is being carried out in the same way by all members of the laboratory staff. That procedure should be one of the two methods outlined in Chapter 14. Second, it is assumed that only meaningful microbial isolates are being tested against relevant antimicrobics; otherwise, exhaustive quality-control efforts are totally meaningless.

Four separate aspects of the standard disc diffusion methods may be identified clearly as being incompletely controlled sources of variability. Each aspect should be monitored independently as part of a regular quality-control program. They are:

1. *Variability in the Actual Potency of the Discs*. Although the FDA currently certifies the potency of all antibiotic discs before they are released for distribution

and sale, discs containing non-antibiotic agents are not certified, and unreliable products are occasionally marketed.[11] In practice, most commercially available discs are reasonably reliable and are not a major source of error. However, discs containing the more labile drugs may lose their potency in transit or while being stored in the clinical laboratory. Proper precautions must be taken to control the environment in which these discs are stored,[8,9] particularly in the smaller laboratory, where discs are likely to be stored for rather long periods of time. An effective quality-control program should monitor the potency of the discs as they are being used.

2. *Variability in Mueller-Hinton Agar.* At the present time, the Mueller-Hinton medium that is being supplied by all the media manufacturers of this country does not perform in an acceptably consistent manner.[3,7,10] Different batches of Mueller-Hinton agar prepared from the same lot can be very reproducible and different lots of medium obtained from the same manufacturer are usually capable of yielding consistent results. This suggests that it is possible to manufacture a consistently reproducible medium for susceptibility testing if the criteria for its preparation are critically defined and carefully followed. Clearly, differences in manufacturing practices may provide agar media that alter the mean zone diameters observed with the control strains.[3,7,10] For proper control, each laboratory must insist upon a single manufacturer as the supplier of its Mueller-Hinton agar, and reasonably large volumes should be purchased, all with the same control number. Each time a new lot of medium is incorporated into a testing program, it should first be tested carefully to be sure that the control limits are the same as with the previous lot. Samples from each batch should also be monitored to detect errors in its preparation and storage.

3. *Variability in Barium-Sulfate Turbidity Standard.* When the standard disc diffusion technique is utilized, the broth cultures are adjusted to match the turbidity of a MacFarland 0.5 turbidity standard. One may anticipate some variability in the actual inoculum attained with different genera.[12] In preparing the barium-sulfate standards, careful attention must be given to the quality of the reagents and to the accuracy of the measurements. The standards may deteriorate on standing unless they are stored in the dark in sealed glass tubes. In practice, it is advisable to replace the turbidity standards at least once every six months, more frequently if controls indicate that something is wrong with the standards.[5] The method by which broth cultures are adjusted to match the $BaSO_4$ standard is actually a much more critical source of variability and must be very carefully standardized and controlled. The need for a $BaSO_4$ turbidity standard is eliminated by the agar overlay method.

4. *Definition of Zone Edge.* With some antimicrobics and certain microorganisms, one often observes rather poorly defined zone edges, and thus the size of the zone actually measured can vary significantly, depending upon the type of light source and the angle of illumination (which should be standardized within each laboratory). Even under well-standardized conditions, there is a degree of subjectivity in selecting the end-point to be measured, and consequently some variability among different persons is to be expected. The definition of the zone edge is markedly improved when test plates are inoculated by the agar overlay technique (Fig. 16-1).

With the standard disc diffusion technique, all four sources of variability must be controlled by carefully standardizing procedures within the laboratory. The performance of the test is then monitored by including standard control strains with each batch of tests. With the agar overlay method, the two sources of error are better controlled; only two critically important sources of variability remain to be monitored on a regular basis—batch-to-batch variability in Mueller-Hinton agar and variability in antimicrobic disc potency.

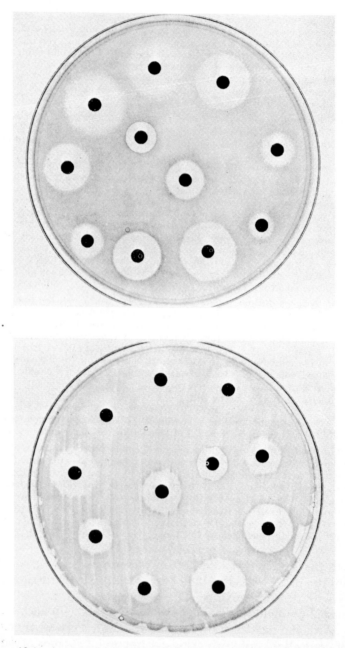

Figure 16-1. Appearance of inhibitory zones (*E. cloacae*) tested with the agar overlay method (*top*) and with the Kirby-Bauer swabbed-plate method (*bottom*). (From A. L. Barry. 1974. In *Current Techniques for Antibiotic Susceptibility Testing.* A. Balows (Ed.). Charles C Thomas, Springfield, Ill. p. 21.)

The performance of the Mueller-Hinton agar can be monitored by testing the standard control strains of *Staphylococcus aureus*, *Escherichia coli* and *Pseudomonas aeruginosa* each time a new batch of plates is prepared. The zones of inhibition should be shown to fall within acceptable limits before the remaining plates from that batch are released for routine use. An effective inventory system must be maintained to be sure that all media are used within one week of preparation unless adequate precautions are taken to minimize evaporation by wrapping in plastic.

Significant variability can result from inactivation of antimicrobic discs during transit or during storage within the laboratory. Exposure to moisture and/or elevated temperatures can alter the activity of antimicrobic discs (especially those containing the penicillins and cephalosporins). The following rapid test system has been developed for monitoring this one important source of variability.

RAPID TEST SYSTEM FOR MONITORING DISC POTENCY

The agar overlay method has been adapted to provide a simple technique for checking the performance of antimicrobic discs just before a batch of tests is to be set up, thus avoiding the delay associated with repeated tests when a cartridge of discs is found to be unsatisfactory.[4] When other controls indicate that difficulties are being encountered, investigations are simplified if it is known that the discs were "in control" at the time that the difficulties were noted. For that reason, routine monitoring of disc potency is very helpful, even though inactive discs are not encountered frequently.

The essential steps involved are outlined in Table 16-1. Once a week, an overnight BHI broth (5-ml) culture is prepared with the control *S. aureus* and *E. coli* stock cultures. Six plates are inoculated with each of the microorganisms. A 0.001-ml calibrated loop is used to seed 9 ml of melted and cooled agar. The seeded agar is then mixed and spread over the surface of a petri plate containing Mueller-Hinton agar randomly sampled from the routine working supply. Up to this point, the technique is identical to the agar overlay method, except that the inoculum is more conveniently prepared by incubating 5 ml of broth overnight. The seeded plates are then allowed to incubate at 35° C for two hours for the *E. coli* and four hours for the *S. aureus*. These pre-incubated plates are then placed in the refrigerator, where they can be held until needed (as long as seven days). Each morning, an inoculated plate is removed from the refrigerator and discs are sampled from the routine laboratory supply. The discs are then applied directly to the cold plates, pressed firmly onto the surface of the agar, and the plates are

Table 16-1. Rapid Test System for Monitoring Disc Potency for Quality Control of Antimicrobic Susceptibility Tests

Once a Week	Each Morning

1. Prepare 16-18 hr. blood agar subculture from stock slants.*
 2. 4-5 colonies to 5 ml BHI, incubate 16-18 hrs. at 35°C.
 3. Inoculate 6 plates each with a 0.001 ml loop, spread in 9 ml of 1.5% agar (as a thin overlay).
 4. Preincubate at 35°C:
    S. aureus   4 hours
    E. coli   2 hours
 5. Refrigerate plates up to 7 days.
	1. Select random sample of discs from working supply.
	 2. Select one *E. coli* and one *S. aureus* plate from refrigerator.
	 3. Apply discs to cold plates.
	 4. Incubate 5 hrs. at 35°C.
	 5. Measure and plot zone diameters. If 2 SD below mean, discard discs and replace from frozen stock supply.

Twice weekly: Test both control strains* with "routine" method, to control media and methods.

Source: A. L. Barry. 1974. In *Current Techniques for Antibiotic Susceptibility Testing*. A. Balows (Ed.). Charles C Thomas, Springfield, Ill. p. 23.
* *E. coli* ATCC 25922 and *S. aureus* ATCC 25923 held on trypticase soy agar slants with weekly transfers and monthly replacement from stock supply stored at −60°C in 15% glycerol broth.

allowed to incubate for five hours at 35° C. At that time, zones of inhibition are just discernible and can be measured if examined with an appropriate light source.

Because the zones of inhibition are a little more difficult to visualize, the rapid test system is not quite as reproducible as the standard methods, which require an overnight period of incubation. However, an overall coefficient of variation of from 5%-10% is easily obtained with either type of procedure. As might be expected, the rapid control test, which involves a period of pre-incubation, gives significantly smaller zones of inhibition than those observed with either of the standard diffusion methods. Thus, separate control limits must be established for the two types of procedures.

In summary, a sample of antimicrobic discs may be selected from the routine working supply each morning for testing with the rapid control technique and the sizes of the zones of inhibition may be plotted on a control chart before the day's batch of tests is performed that afternoon. As long as the results fall within the established 95% confidence limits, one may be reassured that the discs used on that day are capable of performing satisfactorily.

In addition, each time a new batch of Mueller-Hinton agar is prepared, the control *E. coli* and *S. aureus* are tested using the routine procedure. Every three months the zone-size data are reexamined, and for each antimicrobic the mean and standard deviation is calculated for use during the following quarter.

LIMITS OF VARIABILITY PERMISSIBLE WITH CONTROL STRAINS

To control the precision and accuracy of the disc diffusion test the "Seattle" strains of *S. aureus* (ATCC 25923) and *E. Coli* (ATCC 25922) have been designated as standard control organisms and should be included with each day's batch of tests, especially if the standard Kirby-Bauer technique is being used. A gentamicin- and carbenicillin-susceptible strain of *P. aeruginosa* should also be used; the "Boston strain" of *P. aeruginosa* (ATCC 27853) is being recommended for this purpose.[15]

Regular tests should be made with the quality-control strains, and the actual zone of inhibition measured to the nearest whole millimeter and plotted on an easily accessible, easily readable chart.[6] Adequate precision and accuracy in this procedure can be determined by standard statistical methods (95% of the zones should be within 2 SD above or below the mean). Within any given laboratory, zone diameters will vary from day to day over a narrow range—smaller than could be expected if one were to compare zone diameters observed in a number of different laboratories. The FDA has established tolerance limits within which individual control tests should fall if the technique is being performed adequately. The maximal and minimal zone diameters that should be expected with the standard *S. aureus* and *E. coli* strains are listed in Table 16-2. These tolerance limits represent data accumulated from a large number of institutions, and therefore the limits are rather broad.

Ideally, each laboratory should establish its own means and standard deviations every three to six months. The range represented by the mean ± 2 SD should fall within the tolerance limits in Table 16-2. If the means obtained with all or most antimicrobics fall consistently above those listed in Table 16-2, it is probable that the inoculum is too light. Consistently smaller zones suggest excessively heavy inoculum. Declining zone sizes with one of the penicillins or cephalosporins suggest disc deterioration. Divergent results between the aminocyclitols and the tetracyclines suggest that the pH of the medium is incorrectly controlled.

Table 16-2 also lists the maximal standard deviation that could be tolerated on theoretical grounds. These values are based on the differences between the minimal zone size for susceptible strains and the maximal zone size for resistant strains, and they assume that

Table 16-2. Range of Zone Sizes with Individual Values and Theoretical Maximum Standard Deviation Permissible with Standard Control Organisms.

Antimicrobic (high content discs)	E. Coli (ATCC 25922)			S. aureus (ATCC 25923)		
	Mean*	Zone Limits*	Max.SD†	Mean*	Zone Limits*	Max.SD†
Penicillin G	—	—	—	31.5	26–37	2.9
Ampicillin	17.5	15–20	1.3	29.5	24–35	2.9
Carbenicillin‡	23.5	21–26	1.6	—	—	—
Methicillin	—	—	—	19.5	17–22	1.6
Cephalothin	20.5	18–23	1.3	31.0	25–37	1.3
Chloramphenicol	24.0	21–27	1.9	22.5	19–26	1.9
Tetracycline	21.5	18–25	1.6	23.5	19–28	1.6
Erythromycin	11.0	8–14	1.6	26.0	22–30	1.6
Clindamycin	—	—	—	26.0	23–29	1.6
Kanamycin	21.0	17–25	1.6	22.5	19–26	1.6
Streptomycin	16.0	12–20	1.3	18.0	14–22	1.3
Gentamicin	22.5	19–26	1.3	23.0	19–27	1.3
Vancomycin	—	—	—	17.0	15–19	1.3
Polymyxin B	14.0	12–16	1.3	10.0	7–13	1.3
Colistin	13.0	11–15	1.3	—	—	—
Trimethoprim-sulfamethoxazole	29.0	25–33	1.9	28.0	25–31	1.9

* Tolerance limits based on data from FDA collaborative studies and NCCLS standards.

† Theoretical maximum standard deviation permissible without altering the interpretation of the test significantly (P < 0.01), based on the minimum change in zone size that would be required to alter the interpretation from susceptible to resistant. Gentamicin values based on the NCCLS tentative standards of susceptible ≤ 12 mm, resistant ≥ 15 mm.

‡ Data for 50 µg discs, with 100 µg discs, the zone limits and the mean zone should be increased by adding 3 mm. With P. aeruginosa (ATCC 27853) the range is 17 to 21 mm for 50 mcg carbenicillin discs and 20-24 mm for 100 mcg carbenicillin discs.

the standard deviations with clinical isolates would be those of the control organism. If the maximal values are not exceeded, inherent test variables result in a serious interpretive error no more than once in every 100 tests with those strains that give zones just at the interpretive breakpoints. That is to say, the interpretation may vary between resistant and intermediate or between susceptible and intermediate but very rarely between resistant and susceptible. If these control limits are exceeded, there is a significant probability that technical errors are sufficient to result in clinically significant misinterpretations with some of the test microorganisms. The various sources of technical error must then be investigated and corrected when the controls indicate unsatisfactory written results.

OTHER SOURCES OF ERROR

Common sources of error which are not eradicated by testing standard strains include typographical errors in recording the results and technical errors in performing the tests. Many such errors with individual reports often can be detected by reviewing the reports before they are issued and by checking any unusual susceptibility patterns. Certain genera are known to be variable in their susceptibility to some drugs and predictably susceptible or resistant to others. Unusual susceptibility patterns are often traced to an error in the identification of the microorganism or to a technical error in the testing procedure. Thus the susceptibility test can be used as an aid in checking the identification of an individual isolate. Unusual patterns of resistance should be reported only after the culture is checked for purity and the identification is confirmed; occasionally, the susceptibility test should be repeated. Such a practice should be considered an important part of a quality-control program. Petralli et al.[14] recently reported an attempt to put this approach to quality control on a formal basis, incorporating use of an on-line computer to screen the actual zone-size measurements before the test report leaves the laboratory. Such a formal program would certainly be worthy of further trial in those laboratories possessing the necessary facility. With regular monitoring of the test results, the technologists soon become aware of the susceptibility patterns typically seen for different common genera encountered within their institutions.[13]

In conclusion, a thoughtfully planned combination of quality-control procedures can provide a maximum of security with a minimum of effort. As long as the zone diameters observed with the standard control strains fall within the established 95% confidence limits, the major components of the test system are under control. If

Table 16-3. Control Limits for Monitoring Precision and Accuracy of Inhibitory Zone Diameters (mm) Obtained in Groups of Five Separate Observations

Antimicrobic Agent	E. coli (ATCC 25922)			S. aureus (ATCC 25923)		
	Accuracy Control Zone Diameter (mm) Mean of 5 Values	Precision Control Range* of 5 Values Maximum	Average†	Accuracy Control Zone Diameter (mm) Mean of 5 Values	Precision Control Range* of 5 Values Maximum	Average†
Penicillin G	—	—	—	27.8–35.2	13	6.4
Ampicillin	15.8–19.2	6	2.9	25.8–33.2	13	6.4
Methicillin	—	—	—	17.8–21.2	6	2.9
Cephalothin	18.8–22.2	6	2.9	27.0–35.0	14	7.0
Chloramphenicol	22.0–26.0	7	3.5	20.2–24.8	8	4.1
Tetracycline	19.2–23.8	8	4.1	20.5–26.5	11	5.2
Erythromycin	9.0–13.0	7	3.5	23.3–28.7	9	4.7
Clindamycin	—	—	—	24.0–28.0	7	3.5
Kanamycin	18.3–23.7	9	4.7	20.2–24.8	8	4.1
Streptomycin	13.3–18.7	9	4.7	15.3–20.7	9	4.7
Gentamicin	20.2–24.8	8	4.1	20.3–25.7	9	4.7
Vancomycin	—	—	—	15.7–18.3	4	2.3
Polymyxin B	12.7–15.3	4	2.3	—	—	—
Colistin	11.7–14.3	4	2.3	—	—	—
Trimethoprim-sulfamethoxazole	25.3–30.7	9	4.7	25.0–29.0	7	3.5

* Maximum value minus minimum value obtained in a series of five consecutive tests should not exceed the listed maximum limit. The mean should fall within the range listed under "accuracy control."

† In a continuing series of ranges from consecutive groups of five tests each, the average should approximate the listed value.

efforts are also made to check the purity and identification of each of the individual isolates being tested, one may report the results of susceptibility tests with a high degree of confidence.

The control limits listed in Table 16-3 permit precise and accurate monitoring with a minimum of computation. Zone diameters are grouped in sets of five sequentially observed values per set, i.e., from Monday through Friday. Precision (reproducibility) is monitored by means of the range (maximum zone minus minimum zone) within each set of five determinations. The integer value of this range should not exceed the maximum value listed in Table 16-3, and in a continuing series of ranges the collective mean range should come to approximate the listed average range. Accuracy is monitored by comparing the mean zone diameter for each set of five with the range of zone diameter mean values listed in Table 16-3 for each antimicrobic-microorganism combination. If the mean (or range) of the control data exceeds the values listed in Table 16-3, one should suspect that technical systematic error (variation) exists. In that case, the testing procedures should be investigated and corrective action taken.

Common Sources of Error. Although the disc diffusion method is a fairly forgiving procedure, technical errors can compromise accuracy and precision, and one error may either neutralize or compound another type of error. When the controls suggest that the procedure should be reviewed, the following sources of error are commonly discovered:

1. Improper preparation of Mueller-Hinton medium
2. Outdated or improperly stored plates
3. Improperly stored or outdated discs
4. Inadequately standardized inocula
5. Inaccurate preparation or storage of turbidity reference standard
6. Failure to express surplus fluid from the swab before inoculation of plates
7. Excess delay between culture standardization and plate inoculation
8. Excess delay in applying discs after inoculation of plates
9. Delay in incubating plates after applying discs
10. Incubation at temperatures other than 35° C or use of an increased CO_2 atmosphere
11. Premature reading of the test plates before the full 16 to 18 hours
12. Failure to measure zone borders carefully
13. Attempts to test mixed cultures
14. Attempts to test slow-growing strains
15. Transcription errors in recording results of individual tests

REFERENCES

1. Barry, A. L. 1974. The agar overlay technique for disc susceptibility testing. In *Current Techniques for Antibiotic Susceptibility Testing.* A. Balows (Ed.) Charles C Thomas, Springfield, Ill. pp. 17-25.
2. Barry, A. L. 1974. The role of NCCLS in standardization of antimicrobic suscep-

tibility techniques. In *Current Techniques for Antibiotic Susceptibility Testing*. A. Balows (Ed.) Charles C Thomas, Springfield, Ill. pp. 47-53.

3. Barry, A. L., and L. J. Effinger. 1974. Performances of Mueller-Hinton agars prepared by three manufacturers. Am. J. Clin. Pathol. 62:113-117.

4. Barry, A. L., G. D. Fay, and F. W. Atchison. 1972. Quality control of antimicrobial disc susceptibility testing with a rapid method compared to the standard methods. Antimicrob. Agents Chemother. 2:419-422.

5. Bartlett, R. C., and M. Mazens. 1973. Analytical variability in the single disk antimicrobial susceptibility test. Am. J. Clin. Pathol. 59:376-383.

6. Blazovic, D. M., H. Koepcke, and J. M. Matsen. 1971. Quality control testing with the disk antibiotic susceptibility test of Bauer-Kirby-Sherris-Turck. Am. J. Clin. Pathol. 57:592-597.

7. Brenner, V. C., and J. C. Sherris. 1972. Influence of different media and bloods on the results of diffusion antibiotic susceptibility tests. Antimicrob. Agents Chemother. 1:116-122.

8. Griffith, L. J. 1973. *Pseudomonas* resistance due to inactivated susceptibility disks. Antimicrob. Agents Chemother. 4:646-647.

9. Griffith, L. J., and C. G. Mullins. 1968. Drug resistance as influenced by inactivated sensitivity discs. Appl. Microbiol. 16:656-658.

10. Heinze, P., M. Pezzlo, R. Scheir, P. Valter, and L. Thrupp. 1974. Marked effect of commercial media source on standardized susceptibility test results in the clinical laboratory. In abstracts presented at the *14th Interscience Conference on Antimicrobial Agents and Chemotherapy*. American Society for Microbiology, Washington, D. C. Abstract No. 355.

11. Hoo, R., and W. L. Drew. 1974. Potential unreliability of nitrofurantoin disks in susceptibility testing. Antimicrob. Agents Chemother. 5:607-610.

12. Matsen, J. M., M. E. Lund, and D. C. Brooker. 1974. Comparison and evaluation of carbenicillin disks in diffusion susceptibility testing. Antimicrob. Agents Chemother. 5:599-606.

13. O'Brien, T. F., R. L. Kent, and A. A. Medeiras. 1969. Computer-generated plots of results of antimicrobial susceptibility tests. J.A.M.A. 210:84-92.

14. Petralli, J., E. Russell, A. Kataoka, and T. G. Merigan. 1970. On-line computer quality control of antibiotic-sensitivity testing. N. Engl. J. Med. 283:735-738.

15. Reller, L. B., F. D. Schoenknecht, M. A. Kenny, and J. C. Sherris. 1974. Antibiotic susceptibility testing of *Pseudomonas aeruginosa*: Selection of a control strain and criteria for magnesium and calcium content of media. J. Infect. Dis. 130:454-463.

ADDITIONAL REFERENCES

1. Barry, A. L., and R. E. Badal. 1976. Reliability of the microdilution technique for detection of methicillin-resistant strains of *Staphylococcus aureus*. Am. J. Clin. Pathol. (in press).
2. Barry, A. L., L. J. Effinger, and R. E. Badal. 1976. Short-term storage of six penicillins and cephalothin in microdilution trays for antimicrobic susceptibility tests. Antimicrob. Agents Chemother. (in press).
3. Barry, A. L., and R. A. Lasner. 1976. Inhibition of bacterial growth by the nitrofurantoin solvent dimethylformamide. Antimicrob. Agents Chemother. 9:549-550.
4. Blackwell, C. C., and D. S. Feingold. 1975. Frequency and some properties of clinical isolates of methicillin-resistant *Staphylococcus aureus*. Am. J. Clin. Pathol. 64:372-377.
5. Borchardt, K. A. 1976. Laboratory evaluation of a commercial microbial control system. Antimicrob. Agents Chemother. 9:771-775.
6. D'Agostino, R. L., and R. C. Tilton. 1976. Quantitative antibiotic susceptibility testing: *Haemophilus influenzae* type B. Ann. Clin. Lab. Sci. 6: 104-109.
7. Ellner, P. D., and E. Johnson. 1976. Unreliability of direct antibiotic susceptibility testing on wound exudates. Antimicrob. Agents Chemother. 9:355-356.
8. Escamilla, J. 1976. Susceptibility of *Hemophilus influenzae* to ampicillin as determined by use of a modified one-minute beta-lactamase test. Antimicrob. Agents Chemother. 9:196-198.
9. Fass, R. J., R. B. Prior, and C. A. Rotilie. 1975. Simplified method for antimicrobial susceptibility testing of anaerobic bacteria. Antimicrob. Agents Chemother. 8:444-452.
10. Hollick, G. E., and J. A. Washington. 1976. Comparison of direct and standardized disk diffusion susceptibility testing of urine cultures. Antimicrob. Agents Chemother. 9:804-809.
11. Jorgensen, J. H., and J. C. Lee. 1975. Microdilution technique for antimicrobial susceptibility testing of *Haemophilus influenzae*. Antimicrob. Agents Chemother. 8:610-611.
12. Kluge, R. M. 1975. Accuracy of Kirby-Bauer susceptibility tests read at 1, 8, and 12 hours of incubation: Comparison with readings at 18 to 20 hours. Antimicrob. Agents Chemother. 8:139-145.
13. Kunz, L. J., and R. C. Moellering. 1971. Mechanical method of inoculating plates for antibiotic sensitivity testing. Appl. Microbiol. 22:476-477.
14. Lampe, M. F., C. L. Aitken, P. G. Dennis, P. S. Forsythe, K. E. Patrick, F. D. Schoenknecht, and J. C. Sherris. 1975. Relationship of early readings of minimal inhibitory concentrations to the results of overnight tests. Antimicrob. Agents Chemother. 8:429-433.
15. Marks, M. I., and G. Weinmaster. 1975. Influences of media and inocula on the *in vitro* susceptibility of *Haemophilus influenzae* to co-trimoxazole, ampicillin, penicillin, and chloramphenicol. Antimicrob. Agents Chemother. 8:657-663.
16. Pfeiffer, R. R., G. L. Engel, and D. Coleman. 1976. Stable antibiotic sensitivity disks. Antimicrob. Agents Chemother. 9:848-851.
17. Snyder, R. J., P. C. Kohner, D. M. Ilstrup, and J. A. Washington, II. 1976. Analysis of certain variables in the agar dilution susceptibility test. Antimicrob. Agents Chemother. 9:74-76.
18. Washington, J. A., R. J. Snyder, and P. C. Kohner. 1976. Spurious ampicillin resistance by testing *Haemophilus influenzae* with agar containing supplement C. Antimicrob. Agents Chemother. 9:199-200.
19. Wegner, D. L., C. R. Mathis, and T. R. Neblett. 1976. Direct method to determine the antibiotic susceptibility of rapidly growing blood pathogens. Antimicrob. Agents Chemother. 9: 861-862.

INDEX

Page numbers in *italics* refer to illustrations; page numbers followed by t refer to tables.

Hemophilus influenzae, antimicrobic susceptibility of, 84-86
microdilution procedures for, 98-99
minimal inhibitory concentrations with, 20t, 188t
correlates for, 188t
zone-diameter interpretative standards for, 188t
Host factors, influence of, in antimicrobic chemotherapy, 13-15

ICS. *See* International Collaborative Study
Imidazole, activity spectrum of, 32t
molecular weight of, 32t
Incubation, errors in, 119
in agar diffusion tests, 184, 185
in agar dilution technique, 82, 119
in agar overlay method, 185
in anaerobic bacteria testing, 88
in Autobac I test system, 137-138
in disc potency monitoring, 211-212, 212t
in macrodilution procedures, 95
in *Mycobacterium* testing, 159
in *Neisseria gonorrhoeae* testing, 84
in *Staphylococcus aureus* testing, 90, 177
in yeast testing, 150-151
of microdilution trays, 97-98
temperature of, zone of inhibition and, 176-177
time of, zone of inhibition and, 178
Indifference, definition of, 105
determination of, by agar diffusion techniques, 106, *106*
by comparison of killing rates, 112-113, *112*
Infection, as factor in antimicrobic chemotherapy, 14
urinary tract, range of test concentrations for, 70-71
therapy of, 18
INH. *See* Isonicotinic acid hydrazide
Inhibition, zone of. *See* Zone of inhibition
Inhomogeneity of inoculum, 8-9
Inoculation, direct, precautions for, 191-193
errors during, 119
in anaerobic bacteria testing, 88
in disc potency monitoring, 211, 212t
in *Hemophilus influenzae* testing, 85, 86
in macrodilution procedures, 95
in *Mycobacterium* testing, 156
in *Neisseria gonorrhoeae* testing, 84

Inoculation—*Continued*
in yeast testing, 152
methods of, comparison of, 192-193, 192t
of microdilution trays, 97
of test plates, 80-82
overlay method of, 185
standard method of, 7, 184, 191
Inoculum, 10
anaerobe, 98
application of, to agar plates, 80-81
broth cultures of, 72, 80
density of, 72-74, 74t, 80, 97, 124
minimal inhibitory concentrations and, 22-23, 23, 24
zone of inhibition and, 173, 175-176
dilution of, 73-74
direct colony suspension of, 72
for agar dilution techniques, 80
for macrodilution procedures, 93, 95, 98
for microdilution procedures, 95-96, 98-99
Hemophilus influenzae, 85, 98-99
inhomogeneity of, 8-9
Mycobacterium 157-158, 159
Neisseria gonorrhoeae, 83-84
preparation of, 10, 72, 80
quality control of, 124
size of. *See* Inoculum, density of
standardization of, 72-74, 74t, 80, 97
errors in, 118
yeast, 147-148, 150, 152
Inoculum replicator, 80-81, *81*
for microdilution procedures, 97
International Collaborative Study, four-category system of, 25-26
interpretation by, 26t
standard reference methods of, 6-7
Iodometric methods, detection of penicillin β-lactamase activity with, 131
Isobologram, 110-111, *110*
Isolates, anaerobic bacteria, 87
Neisseria gonorrhoeae, storage of, 83
single colony vs. mixed culture, 10
Isoniazid, diluent for, 70t
distribution of, in *Mycobacterium* testing, 158t
peak serum concentration of, 17t
solvent for, 70t
Isonicotinic acid hydrazide, activity spectrum of, 32t
molecular weight of, 32t
properties of, 41-42
structural formula for, *42*